For Butterworth-Heinemann:

Senior Commissioning Editor: Mary Seager
Development Editor: Catharine Steers
Project Managers: Pat Miller; Gail Wright
Designer: Andy Chapman
Illustrations Manager: Bruce Hogarth
Page Layout: Jim Hope (Publishing Technology Unit, Elsevier)

Introduction to Veterinary Anatomy and Physiology

Victoria Aspinall BVSc MRCVS

Principal, Abbeydale Veterinary Training,
Gloucester, UK

Melanie O'Reilly BSc(Hons) Zoology PGCE VN

Lecturer, College of Animal Welfare,
Potters Bar, London, UK

Foreword by

Andrea Jeffery CertEd DipAVN(Surg) VN

Tutor in Veterinary Nursing,
Department of Clinical Veterinary Science,
University of Bristol, Bristol, UK

Illustrations by
Antbits Illustration
Saffron Walden, UK

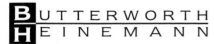

BUTTERWORTH
HEINEMANN

An imprint of Elsevier

Edinburgh • London • New York • Oxford • Philadelphia • St Louis • Sydney • Toronto 2004

Butterworth-Heinemann
An imprint of Elsevier Limited

First published 2004
  Reprinted 2005 (twice), 2006, 2007 (twice), 2008

ISBN-13: 978–0–7506–8782–9

British Library Cataloguing in Publication Data
A catalogue record for this book is available from the British Library

Library of Congress Cataloging in Publication Data
A catalog record for this book is available from the Library of Congress

Notice
Veterinary knowledge is constantly changing. Standard safety precautions must be followed, but as
new research and clinical experience broaden our knowledge, changes in treatment and drug therapy
may become necessary or appropriate. Readers are advised to check the most current product
information provided by the manufacturer of each drug to be administered to verify the
recommended dose, the method and duration of administration, and contraindications. It is the
responsibility of the practitioner, relying on experience and knowledge of the patient, to determine
dosages and the best treatment for each individual patient. Neither the Publisher nor the authors
assume any liability for any injury and/or damage to persons or property arising from
this publication.

The Publisher

The
publisher's
policy is to use
**paper manufactured
from sustainable forests**

Printed in China

CONTENTS

Foreword vii
Preface ix
About the authors x
Acknowledgements xi

Section 1 – The dog and cat

1. Principles of Cell Biology 3
2. Tissues and Body Cavities 17
3. Skeletal System 27
4. Muscular System 45
5. Nervous System and Special Senses 56
6. Endocrine System 77
7. Blood Vascular System 84
8. Respiratory System 98
9. Digestive System 107
10. Urinary System 122
11. Reproductive System 134
12. Common Integument 151

Section 2 – Exotic species

13. Birds 159
14. Mammals 173
15. Reptiles and fish 190

References and recommended reading 204
Appendix 1 – Introduction to anatomical terminology 207
Appendix 2 – Multiple Choice Questions 209
          Multiple Choice Answers 224
Index 225

FOREWORD

The continued advancement of the role of the veterinary nurse in veterinary practice necessitates a thorough education and training. This book will support students during their studies. It is an eminently suitable text for certificate and undergraduate level nurses as well as a useful revision aid for those embarking on their Diploma.

One very important feature of the book is that it clearly relates the anatomy and physiology to clinical cases seen within practice, which will enable veterinary nursing students to see the relevance of the subject that they are being taught as it puts it into a clinical context.

The authors have presented the information using a variety of methods including text, bullet points, tables, and clearly labelled diagrams and radiographs supporting the main part of the text. There is a continuity of style throughout the book with the use of italics highlighting key words within the text and a 'key points' section at the end of each chapter. A useful MCQ self-test appendix will enable students to check their learning.

I congratulate the authors on writing this Introduction to Veterinary Anatomy and Physiology, as it is a timely addition to the veterinary textbooks currently available. I am sure that nurses will remember this as the textbook that helped them succeed in their anatomy and physiology examinations.

Bristol 2003   *Andrea Jeffery*

PREFACE

Introduction to Veterinary Anatomy and Physiology is intended as a foundation text for a subject that underpins everything that is done in veterinary practice. It is designed for students who have studied biological science at GCSE and who want to increase their depth of understanding and apply the knowledge to companion animals. The authors anticipate that its principal use will be to student veterinary nurses preparing for their professional exams and the text is largely based on the veterinary nursing objective syllabus; however, the inclusion of a wider range of species will also make it of interest to students of animal science both at National Diploma and degree levels. It may even be useful to veterinary students who need to make the leap from their A-levels, based on human anatomy and physiology, to the first year of a course that is based entirely on animals.

The book is divided into two main sections. Section 1 provides detailed description of the anatomy and physiology of the dog and the cat while Section 2 builds on the basic plan to cover more exotic species, including birds, small rodents, reptiles and fish. These animals are becoming more and more popular as pets and an understanding of their anatomy and physiology is fundamental to the development of care systems. The whole text is supplemented by large numbers of clear diagrams that help the student to understand the concepts being described.

Scattered throughout the text, fragments identified as 'Applied Anatomy' relate the anatomical facts to veterinary disease conditions, the nursing protocols commonly used in veterinary practice and, in some cases, to useful pieces of information that make the study of the animal world even more fascinating. These should help the student veterinary nurse to understand why the study of anatomy and physiology is so important to the job of a veterinary nurse.

The authors have long felt that there is a need for a good basic anatomy and physiology textbook based on the species seen in small animal practice and hope that this book will fulfil that niche.

Victoria Aspinall
Melanie O'Reilly

Gloucester and Potters Bar 2003

ABOUT THE AUTHORS

Victoria Aspinall BVSc MRCVS qualified from Bristol University in 1974 and went into small animal practice in Kings Lynn, Norfolk with her husband, who is also a vet. After five years, including brief spells in practices in Sussex and Swindon, they set up a small animal practice in Gloucester. In 1991 Vicky was employed to help start the new Animal Care department at Hartpury College, Gloucester, and in 1993 was appointed Head of Animal Care and Veterinary Nursing. In 1999 she started Abbeydale Veterinary Training above her husband's practice and is now a director of Abbeydale Vetlink Veterinary Training Ltd. Vicky has contributed to *Veterinary Nursing Journal*, has been responsible for a series of CD-Roms on anatomy and physiology and has written chapters in *Pre-Veterinary Nursing Textbook* (Masters & Bowden), *Textbook of Veterinary Medical Nursing* (Bowden & Masters) and *Veterinary Nursing*, Third Edition (Lane & Cooper). She has recently edited *Clinical Procedures for Veterinary Nurses*. Vicky has four children – none of whom wishes to follow their parents into the profession!

Melanie O'Reilly BSc(Hons) Zoology PGCE VN qualified in 1990 and worked at the Royal Veterinary College. During that time, she attended evening classes to take the necessary A-levels in order to fulfil her ambition of studying zoology. In 1993 she gained a place at London University and graduated with honours three years later. Her final-year dissertation on wolf behaviour allowed her to carry out a behavioural study on the wolf pack at Whipsnade. In 1998, after taking a break to start a family, Melanie began teaching student veterinary nurses at the College of Animal Welfare and now lectures in anatomy and physiology at the CAW's Royal Veterinary College site. She has written a chapter on the evolution of the wolf and the domestication of the dog for the *Ultimate Dog Care Book* and has recently co-authored (with Vicky Aspinall) the chapter on anatomy and physiology in the new edition of *Veterinary Nursing*.

ACKNOWLEDGEMENTS

The completion of this book would not have been possible without the support of all the members of our respective families, including Richard, Polly, Charlie, William, Nico, Evelyn, Ken, Sebastian, Elizabeth and Rodolfo, who put up with starvation and neglect, obsession with hitting deadlines, and our grumpiness!

We would also like to thank the many colleagues who have lent us material, in particular Neil Forbes, Greg Simpson and Mike Daly for the loan of some very useful books. Finally, we are grateful to Mary Seager and Barbara Cooper for their faith that we could write this book and to Catharine Steers and Gail Wright at Elsevier, who are always willing to sympathise and rearrange dates when life interferes with the grand plan.

SECTION

1

THE DOG AND CAT

1   Principles of Cell Biology *3*

2   The Tissues and Body Cavities *17*

3   The Skeletal System *27*

4   The Muscular System *45*

5   The Nervous System and Special Senses *56*

6   The Endocrine System *77*

7   The Blood Vascular System *84*

8   The Respiratory System *100*

9   The Digestive System *109*

10 The Urinary System *124*

11 The Reproductive System *136*

12 The Common Integument *153*

This section describes the anatomy and physiology of the two most common species treated in veterinary practice: the dog and cat. Following an introduction to cell biology, each body system is covered separately.

I PRINCIPLES OF CELL BIOLOGY

Anatomy and physiology are scientific terms used to describe the study of the structure of the body (anatomy) and how the body actually 'works' (physiology). In this Section, we will study the anatomy and physiology of the dog and cat. In Section 2, the anatomy and physiology of the exotic species most commonly kept as pets is covered. We start by looking at the basic unit of the body – the cell – and then work our way through the tissues and systems until the picture is complete.

ANIMAL CLASSIFICATION

When studying any aspect of biology it is important to have a basic understanding of the classification system used to group animals. How the species that one may meet in a veterinary practice fit into this classification system should also be understood. Classification is the way in which we 'sort' species into orderly groups, depending on how closely they are related in terms of their evolution, structure and behaviour. The science of classification is known as *taxonomy*.

If organisms have certain basic features in common they are grouped together into a *kingdom*. For example, if an organism is composed of more than one cell, i.e. it is multicellular, and obtains its food by ingestion, it is placed in the animal kingdom. Other kingdoms include plants and fungi. The animal kingdom is then further subdivided, based upon similarities of organisms, into a hierarchical system (Table 1.1). This narrows the classification down until we eventually reach a particular *genus* and *species*. Most living organisms are identified by a genus and species – a method known as the binomial system and invented by the Swedish scientist Carl Linnaeus.

All the species within the animal kingdom are divided into those with backbones – the vertebrates – and those that do not have backbones – the invertebrates, e.g. insects, worms, etc. The vertebrates are divided into eight *classes*. The classes that are of the most veterinary importance are:

- Amphibia – approximately 3080 species
- Reptilia – approximately 6600 species
- Aves or birds – approximately 8500 species
- Fish – approximately 30 000 species.
- Mammalia – approximately 4070 species.

These classes are then further divided into *orders*, and so on, until a species is identified, as in Table 1.1.

Table 1.1 Classification of the domestic dog and cat.		
Taxonomic group	Dog	Cat
Kingdom	Animal	Animal
Phylum	Chordata (Vertebrate)	Chordata (Vertebrate)
Class	Mammalia (Mammal)	Mammalia (Mammal)
Order	Carnivora	Carnivora
Family	Canidae	Felidae
Genus	*Canis*	*Felis*
Species	*familiaris*	*catus*
Common Name	Domestic Dog	Domestic Cat

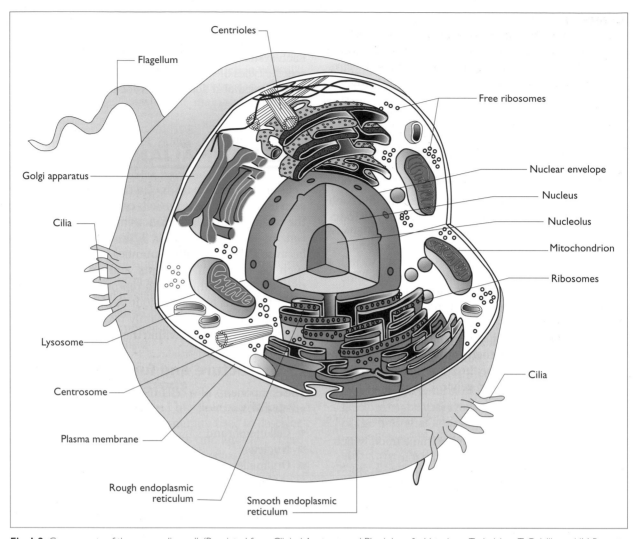

Centrioles

Flagellum

Free ribosomes

Golgi apparatus

Nuclear envelope

Cilia

Nucleus

Nucleolus

Mitochondrion

Ribosomes

Lysosome

Cilia

Centrosome

Plasma membrane

Rough endoplasmic
reticulum

Smooth endoplasmic
reticulum

Fig. 1.2 Components of the mammalian cell. (Reprinted from Clinical Anatomy and Physiology for Veterinary Technicians, T Colville and JM Bassett, p 11, Copyright 2002, with permission from Elsevier Science.)

1. Pores in the cell membrane – small molecules can pass through these pores
2. Simple diffusion – molecules that are soluble in lipids (or fats) will passively dissolve in the lipid part of the cell membrane and diffuse across it; oxygen and water enter the cell in this way

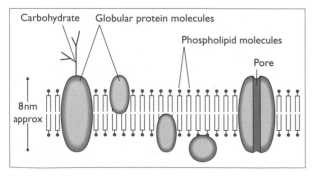

Carbohydrate   Globular protein molecules

Phospholipid molecules

Pore

8nm
approx

Fig. 1.3 Structure of the cell membrane showing the phospholipid bilayer. This structure is also known as the 'fluid mosaic model'.

3. Facilitated diffusion – this is another type of passive diffusion, i.e. where the substance is moving down a concentration gradient, but the substance enlists the help of a carrier protein to help it across the membrane; glucose uses this method to enter the cell
4. Active transport mechanisms – substances are usually being moved from a region of low concentration to one of higher concentration, i.e. they are travelling against a concentration gradient. This is like going up a steep hill – it is hard work and therefore requires energy. Substances that require active transport mechanisms to cross the cell membrane use a carrier protein to transport them across. The 'cost' for this service is that energy is required, and is supplied by the cell's 'energy currency' – molecules of adenosine triphosphate or ATP. Sodium enters the cell this way.

Cytoplasm

This is the fluid that fills the interior of the cell, providing it with support. The nucleus and organelles are found within the cytoplasm, along with solutes such as glucose, proteins and ions.

Nucleus

The nucleus is the information centre of the cell. It is surrounded by a nuclear membrane and contains the *chromosomes*. Chromosomes are the bearers of the hereditary material, DNA, which carries the information for protein synthesis. DNA is the 'set of instructions' that tells the cell how to function, and these instructions are then passed on to the cell's descendents. The nucleus also contains several nucleoli, where the ribosomes (see below) are manufactured.

Organelles

1. *Mitochondria* – these are responsible for cellular respiration and are the site where energy is extracted from food substances and stored in a form that the cell can use: adenosine triphosphate or ATP. Mitochondria have a smooth outer membrane and a highly folded inner membrane, which increases the surface area on which ATP production can take place (Fig. 1.2). Mitochondria are found in abundance in cells that are very active in terms of energy consumption, e.g. skeletal muscle. When a cell requires energy it uses its store of ATP molecules. The energy itself is stored in the bond that connects the phosphate group to the rest of the molecule (Fig. 1.4). If one of these phosphate groups is 'snapped off' the molecule, the bond is broken and energy is released. The remaining molecule is now called ADP or adenosine *di*phosphate, because it now has only two phosphate groups attached to it (di = 2; tri = 3). However, the cell needs only to re-attach another phosphate group (carried out as part of the cell's metabolic processes), and energy can be stored once more as ATP.
2. *Ribosomes* – these float free in the cytoplasm and are the site for protein synthesis within the cell.
3. *Endoplasmic reticulum (ER)* – this is a network of membrane-lined interconnected tubes and cavities within the cytoplasm of the cell. There are two types of endoplasmic reticulum:
   - *Rough endoplasmic reticulum* is so called because it has numerous ribosomes attached to its surface and thus appears 'rough' when viewed under a microscope. The function of rough ER is to transport the proteins which have been synthesised by ribosomes. Some of these proteins are not required by the cell in which they are made but are 'exported' outside the cell, e.g. digestive enzymes and hormones.

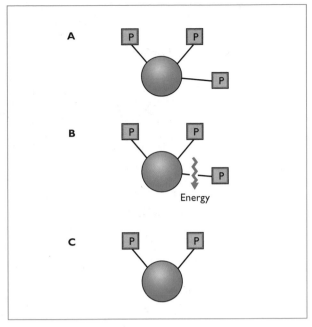

Fig. 1.4 The conversion of ATP to ADP to release energy. A The ATP molecule has three phosphate groups (P) attached by chemical bonds; energy is stored within the bonds. B One of the phosphate groups is 'snapped off', releasing energy. C The remaining molecule (ADP, with two phosphate groups) goes back into the metabolic cycle and has a phosphate group reattached, becoming ATP again.

   - *Smooth endoplasmic reticulum* is so called because it does not have ribosomes on its surface; its functions include the synthesis and transport of lipids and steroids.
4. *The Golgi apparatus* or body – this is a stack of flattened sacs within the cytoplasm (Fig. 1.2). Its function includes the modification of some of the proteins produced by the cell (adding a carbohydrate component) and it plays a part in the formation of lysosomes.
5. *Lysosomes* – these are membrane-bound sacs that contain lysozymes or digestive enzymes. Their function is to digest materials taken in by the cell during the process of phagocytosis or endocytosis (Fig. 1.5). Lysosomes also destroy worn out organelles within the cell and, in some cases, the cell itself.
6. *Centrosome and centrioles* – the centrosome contains a pair of rod-like structures called centrioles. These lie at right angles to each other and are involved in cell division (see mitosis).
7. *Cilia and flagella* – these are extensions of the plasma membrane seen on some cells of the body. Cilia are found in large numbers on the outer surface of the cells and are responsible for creating a wave-like motion which moves fluid

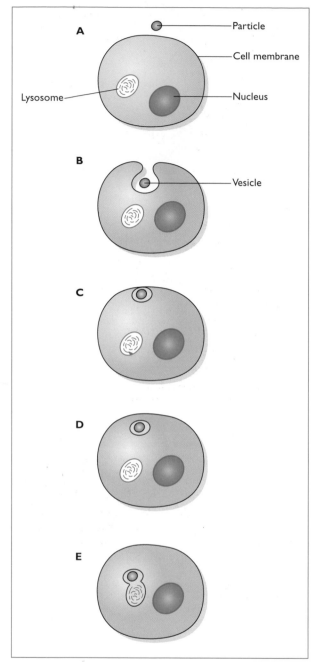

Fig. 1.5 Phagocytosis. **A** A small particle (e.g. bacterium) is present outside the cell. **B** The cell membrane invaginates and starts to enclose the particle. **C** The cell membrane completely surrounds the particle and seals it off in a vesicle. **D** The vesicle detaches from the membrane and enters the cell. **E** A lysosome, containing digestive enzymes, fuses with the phagocytic vesicle containing the particle and the particle is destroyed.

such as mucus and debris over the cell surface. Flagella are usually single and longer than cilia and move the cell along by undulating movements. The only example of a flagellum in mammals is the tail of a spermatozoon.

Materials can either be taken into the cell or exported out of it. These processes are called *endocytosis* and *exocytosis* respectively. There are two types of endocytosis: phagocytosis or 'cell eating' and pinocytosis or 'cell drinking'. During both these processes the cell surface folds to make a small pocket that is lined by the cell membrane (Fig. 1.5). The pocket seals off, forming a vesicle that contains the material being brought into the cell. This separates from the cell surface, moves into the cell's interior and fuses with a lysosome, containing lysozymes, which digest the vesicle contents. The process of phagocytosis is also used to remove foreign particles such as invading bacteria (see blood cells).

Cell division

The cells of the body are classified into two types:

1. *Somatic cells* – these include all the cells of the body except those involved in reproduction. Somatic cells divide by *mitosis* and contain the *diploid number* of chromosomes.
2. *Germ cells* – these are the ova (within the ovaries) and the spermatozoa (within the testes). Germ cells divide by *meiosis* and contain the *haploid number* of chromosomes.

Mitosis

The tissues of the body grow, particularly when the animal is young, and are able to repair themselves when damaged. This is achieved by the process of mitosis in which the somatic cells of the body make identical copies of themselves. The cells replicate by dividing into two – a process called *binary fission*. However, before they can do this they must first make a copy of all the hereditary or genetic information that the new cell will need in order to function normally. This information is carried in the DNA (deoxyribonucleic acid) of the chromosomes within the nucleus of the parent cell. The normal number of chromosomes is described as the diploid number and before cell division takes place the chromosomes are duplicated (Fig. 1.6).

Mitosis can be divided into four active stages, followed by a 'resting' stage (called *interphase*), during which the new daughter cells grow and prepare for the next division. Interphase is not actually a resting stage because it is during this stage that the DNA replicates in preparation for the next mitosis. The centrioles have also replicated by the start of the new mitotic division. The four active stages of mitosis are:

1. *Prophase* – the nuclear membrane breaks down and the chromosomes contract and become shorter, fatter and more distinct. The identical

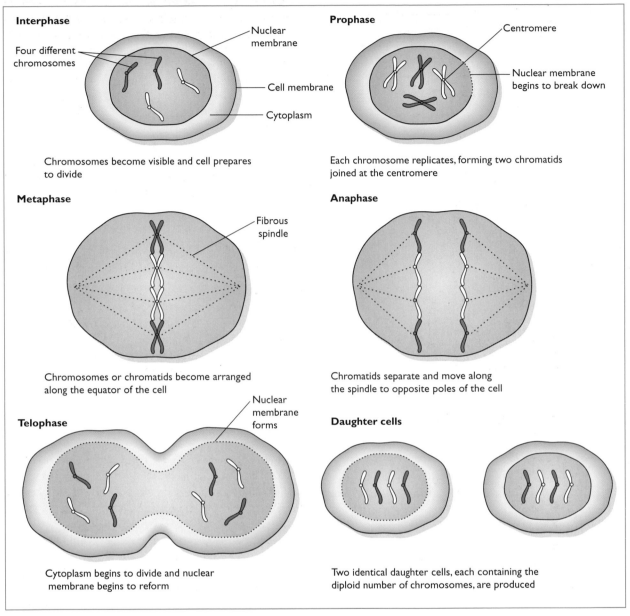

Interphase

Four different chromosomes

Nuclear membrane

Cell membrane

Cytoplasm

Chromosomes become visible and cell prepares to divide

Prophase

Centromere

Nuclear membrane begins to break down

Each chromosome replicates, forming two chromatids joined at the centromere

Metaphase

Fibrous spindle

Chromosomes or chromatids become arranged along the equator of the cell

Anaphase

Chromatids separate and move along the spindle to opposite poles of the cell

Telophase

Nuclear membrane forms

Cytoplasm begins to divide and nuclear membrane begins to reform

Daughter cells

Two identical daughter cells, each containing the diploid number of chromosomes, are produced

Fig. 1.6 Mitosis – the cell division seen in somatic cells.

pairs of chromosomes have not yet separated and are referred to as the *chromatids*. The chromatids are held together at a region called the centromere. The centrioles are now found at the opposite poles or ends of the cell and spindle fibres start to form. These are 'threads' passing from the centriole at one pole to the centriole at the other pole.

2. *Metaphase* – the chromosomes line up in the middle of the cell (known as the equator) and the chromatids draw apart at the centromere.

3. *Anaphase* – the chromosomes attach to the spindle fibres and as these contract it moves the chromatids towards the opposite poles of the cell.

4. *Telophase* – the chromatids will be the chromosomes of the daughter cells. The spindle fibres break down and the nuclear membrane reforms. The cell starts to constrict across the middle and continues until it is divided into two. Each of the new daughter cells is genetically identical to the original parent cell, and both contain the full set of chromosomes, known as the diploid number. The chromosomes then unravel and the cell returns to interphase.

Mitosis results in the production of two identical daughter cells, each of which is identical to the parent cell and contains the diploid number of chromosomes.

Meiosis

This is the process by which the germ cells divide within the ovary of the female and the testis of the male. Meiosis results in the production of ova or sperm containing *half* the normal number of chromosomes (the haploid number). Meiosis must occur before fertil-isation, when a sperm penetrates the ovum and the two nuclei fuse. If those two nuclei had the diploid number of chromosomes then the nucleus of the resulting gamete would have twice the normal number and abnormalities would develop.

The resting cell is in interphase before meiosis begins. The eight stages are as follows (see also Fig. 1.7):

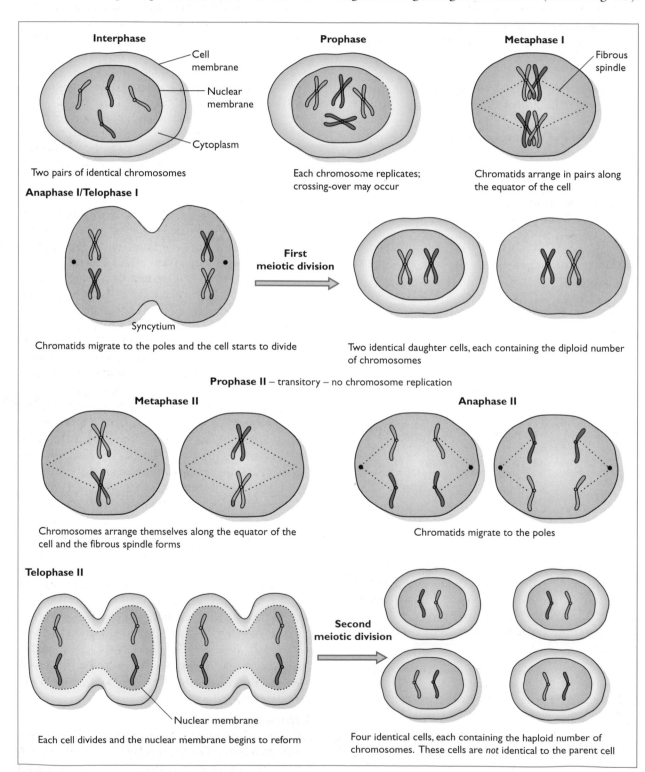

Interphase

Cell membrane

Nuclear membrane

Cytoplasm

Two pairs of identical chromosomes

Prophase

Each chromosome replicates; crossing-over may occur

Metaphase I

Fibrous spindle

Chromatids arrange in pairs along the equator of the cell

Anaphase I/Telophase I

Syncytium

Chromatids migrate to the poles and the cell starts to divide

First meiotic division

Two identical daughter cells, each containing the diploid number of chromosomes

Prophase II – transitory – no chromosome replication

Metaphase II

Chromosomes arrange themselves along the equator of the cell and the fibrous spindle forms

Anaphase II

Chromatids migrate to the poles

Telophase II

Nuclear membrane

Each cell divides and the nuclear membrane begins to reform

Second meiotic division

Four identical cells, each containing the haploid number of chromosomes. These cells are *not* identical to the parent cell

Fig. 1.7 Meiosis – the cell division seen in the germ cells.

1. *Prophase* – this takes longer than prophase in mitosis. The homologous (identical) chromosomes lie side by side and duplicate; each pair is joined at the centromere. These chromosomes may become entangled and pieces of one chromosome may become attached to another – this process is known as 'crossing over' and may influence the characteristics of the offspring.
2. *Metaphase I* – the homologous pairs of chromosomes come to lie along the line of the equator of the cell and the fibrous spindle starts to form.
3. *Anaphase I* – the pairs separate and the chromatids migrate along the spindle fibres towards the poles of the cell.
4. *Telophase I* – the cytoplasm begins to divide but the nuclear membrane does not reform. In some cells, the cytoplasm does not divide completely and a dumb-bell shaped cell is seen – this is known as a *syncytium*. Telophase I is the *first meiotic division*.
5. *Prophase II* – this may be transitory as there is no need to replicate the chromosomes.
6. *Metaphase II* – the chromosomes arrange themselves along the equator and the spindle fibres appear.
7. *Anaphase II* – the chromatids pull apart and migrate towards the poles of the cells.
8. *Telophase II* – the cytoplasm begins to divide, the nuclear membrane reforms and four identical daughter cells are formed. Telophase II is the *second meiotic division*.

Meiosis results in the production of four identical daughter cells, each of which is non-identical to the parent cell and contains the haploid number of chromosomes.

THE CHEMISTRY OF THE BODY

The cells, and therefore the tissues and organs which are all made of cells, are composed of chemicals. It is important to be able to understand these chemicals and the reactions in which they take part within the body. Chemical compounds can be divided into two groups:

- *Organic* compounds are those that contain the element carbon
- *Inorganic* compounds are all those compounds that do not contain carbon.

Both groups are found in the body, but let us first look at the most biologically important inorganic compound of the body – water (H_2O).

Water content of the body

An individual mammalian cell contains approximately 80% water. In fact, 60–70% of the whole body's weight is water, which is divided into two main body compartments: *intracellular* and *extracellular* water.

Intracellular fluid (ICF) is that which is found inside the cells of the body and can be subdivided into the fluid within the blood cells and the fluid in all other cells. ICF takes up 40% of total body weight.

Extracellular fluid (ECF) is that which lies outside the cells, i.e. the surrounding environment of the cells. ECF takes up 20% of total body weight and includes the fluid in which the blood cells are suspended (the plasma), the fluid within the lymphatic system and the cerebrospinal fluid (the transcellular fluid), and the fluid that surrounds all the other cells of the body (the interstitial or tissue fluid).

Plasma takes up about 5% of body weight. It forms the medium in which the blood cells are transported within the blood-vascular system. It is rich in proteins, termed plasma proteins. *Transcellular fluid* is formed by active secretory mechanisms and its volume varies. It is considered to take up about 1% of body weight and it includes fluids such as cerebrospinal fluid, digestive juices and lymph. *Interstitial fluid* takes up 15% of body weight and lies outside the blood vascular system, surrounding the cells. It is formed from the blood by a process of ultrafiltration – small molecules and ions are separated from larger molecules and cells. The pressure in the blood vascular system forces the fluid through the walls of the capillaries. This acts like a sieve, holding back the large plasma protein molecules and the cellular components of the blood, and allowing everything else to go through. Thus, interstitial fluid is similar to plasma but *without* the blood cells and protein molecules. Interstitial fluid is the medium in which the cells are bathed and from it the cells extract all that they need, such as oxygen and nutrients. They get rid of all their unwanted waste products into it.

Water or fluid provides the medium in which all the body's biochemical reactions take place and is thus essential to maintain the body's internal environment in a state of balance – this is a process known as *homeostasis*. Body water and the chemical substances within it constantly move around the body. The biological processes that are responsible for this movement are diffusion and osmosis.

Diffusion (Fig. 1.8A)
Diffusion is the movement of molecules of a liquid or a gas down a concentration gradient, i.e. from a region where they are at a high concentration to a region

where they are at a lower concentration. Diffusion will occur until an equilibrium is reached, i.e. until the concentration equalises out. Diffusion takes place where there is no barrier to the free movement of molecules or ions and is very important in their movement in and out of cells. However, it can only occur if the particle size is small enough to pass through the cell membrane. If the molecules are too large, then another process takes place in order to achieve equilibrium – this is known as osmosis.

Osmosis (Fig. 1.8B)

Osmosis is the movement of water through a *semipermeable membrane* from a fluid of low concentration to one of a higher concentration, which continues until the two concentrations are equal. The water can be considered to be diffusing along a concentration gradient. A semi-permeable membrane allows some substances through but not others. Osmosis is responsible for water movement from the interstitial fluid into the cells.

A solution consists of the molecules of one substance (the solute) dissolved in another substance (the solvent). In the body, the solvent is water so osmosis is a significant factor in the maintenance of the fluid volume within the body fluid compartments. A solution can be described as having an *osmotic pressure*. This is the pressure needed to prevent osmosis from occurring and is dependent on the number of particles, both dissolved and undissolved, in the solution, e.g. if the osmotic pressure of the plasma is high, water will flow into the blood to equalise the concentration; if the

osmotic pressure of the plasma is low, water will flow out of the blood into the tissue spaces.

Fluid balance

Water is constantly moving within the body, e.g. from the interstitial fluid into the cells, from the plasma to the tissue fluid, etc. but it is also continually lost from the body and must be replaced to ensure that the total fluid balance in the body is maintained. Water is lost through the respiratory system (expired air contains water vapour), and in the urine and faeces. Dogs and cats do not sweat appreciably but do lose heat and water through panting. Water is also lost in the tears, which are produced constantly to moisten the eye, and in vaginal secretions. Water is taken into the body

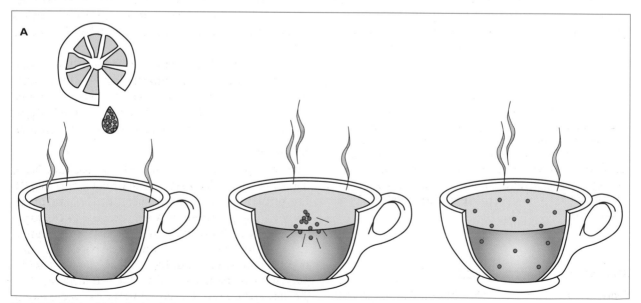

Fig. 1.8A Diffusion. Molecules in solution are active and constantly collide into one another. With time, they become evenly distributed throughout the liquid, having moved down concentration gradients from areas of high concentration to those of low, until equilibrium is reached. Diffusion occurs when there is no barrier to free movement and it occurs more rapidly in hot liquids than in cold ones as molecules are more active at higher temperatures. (Reprinted from Clinical Anatomy and Physiology for Veterinary Technicians, T Colville and JM Bassett, p 24, Copyright 2002, with permission from Elsevier Science.)

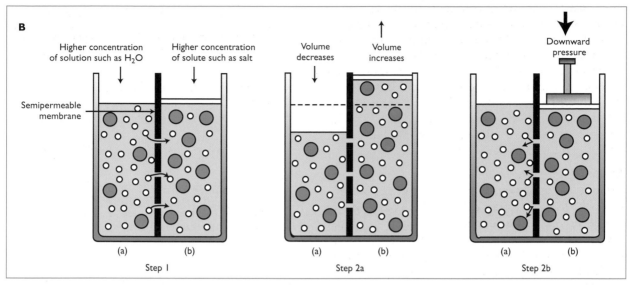

Fig. 1.8B Osmosis. Step 1: Smaller molecules of solution in side (a) can pass through the semi-permeable membrane into side (b), but the larger molecules of solute can not. Step 2a: As solution moves from side (a) to side (b), the volume of side (b) increases until the concentration of solute is the same on both sides. Step 2b: Osmosis can be reversed by filtration, when hydraulic pressure is placed on side (b). This forces solution back through the semi-permeable membrane to side (a). (Reprinted from Clinical Anatomy and Physiology for Veterinary Technicians, T Colville and JM Bassett, p 25, Copyright 2002, with permission from Elsevier Science.)

through drinking fluids and from the water content of food.

Fluid losses may be increased in sick or injured animals, e.g. vomiting, diarrhoea, vaginal discharge (as seen with an open pyometra) or blood loss. This can lead to dehydration, which may cause serious consequences such as reduction of the circulating blood volume, known as hypovolaemic shock. In a normal adult animal, about 60% of the total bodyweight is water. This percentage will be slightly lower if the animal is old or very obese (fatty tissue contains little water) or slightly higher in young or thin animals.

> Typical daily water loss is: 20 mL per kg bodyweight in the urine; 10–20 mL per kg bodyweight in the faeces; and 20 mL per kg bodyweight through the loss of water vapour in expired air and panting and in body secretions – a total of 50–60 mL of water per kg of bodyweight daily. Thus an adult healthy animal should take in 50–60 mL of water per kg bodyweight per day to balance the normal fluid loss, e.g. an animal weighing 20 kg will need 1000–1200 mL of water each day.

Inorganic compounds

There are a number of other inorganic compounds that are also essential to the functions of the body: minerals, acids and bases. It is important to be familiar with some basic chemical definitions when considering these substances. Everything is composed of *atoms*,

and an *element* is a substance that is composed of only one kind of atom, e.g. the element oxygen consists only of oxygen atoms. *Molecules* consist of two or more atoms linked by a chemical bond. A substance whose molecules contain more than one type of atom is called a *compound.*

When dissolved in water, the molecules of many substances break apart into charged particles, called *ions.* This charge may either be negative or positive: ions with one or more positive charges are called *cations* and ions with one or more negative charges are called *anions.*

An *electrolyte* is a chemical substance that, when dissolved in water, splits into ions, and is thus capable of conducting an electric current. Sodium chloride (NaCl) is an example of an electrolyte in the body, its ions being sodium (Na^+) and chloride (Cl^-) in solution.

Minerals

The principal cations in the body are sodium (Na^+), potassium (K^+), calcium (Ca^{2+}), and magnesium (Mg^{2+}). The principal anions include chloride (Cl^-) and bicarbonate (HCO_3^-). These ions are essential to the functions of the body and it is vital that they are present in sufficient and balanced quantities. Sodium and chloride are mainly found in the extracellular fluid, while potassium is mainly found in the intracellular fluid (i.e. inside the cells). The concentration of these ions is important in the regulation of fluid balance between the intracellular and extracellular fluid. This balance is maintained by special 'pumps' in the cell membrane. An imbalance will lead to significant problems, e.g. sodium affects the osmotic pressure of the blood and so influences blood volume and pressure; a high concentration of potassium in the extracellular fluid can disrupt heart function.

Calcium, phosphorus and magnesium are important minerals that are found in storage in bone tissue. Calcium is essential for many processes in the body, such as muscle contraction, nerve conduction and blood clotting. Iron and copper are also essential to normal body function, iron being an essential component of the haemoglobin in red blood cells.

Acids and bases

An *acid* is a compound that can release hydrogen ions when dissolved in solution. Compounds that can accept or take in hydrogen ions are called *bases* or *alkalis*. The acidity of a solution is expressed as its pH, which is the measure of the hydrogen ion concentration. The pH scale is from 0–14, with a pH of 7 being neutral. A solution with a pH less than 7 is acidic (the lower the number the higher the acidity, i.e. the greater the concentration of hydrogen ions). A solution with a pH above 7 is basic or alkaline (the higher the number the more alkaline the solution).

> The pH of body fluids is 7.35 and it is important that the body maintains this level. Within the respiratory system and kidney there are homeostatic processes to maintain the correct acid/base balance.

Organic compounds

These are compounds that are based on the element carbon. The other main elements found in organic compounds are oxygen and hydrogen, and in some instances nitrogen. The principal organic compounds found in the body are carbohydrates, proteins and fats.

Carbohydrates

Carbohydrates contain carbon, hydrogen and oxygen and are also known as sugars. Sugars are an important source of energy and the most common simple sugar in the body is glucose (Fig. 1.9). Simple sugars can join together to form more complex carbohydrates; when many sugars join together they form a *polysaccharide*, e.g. glycogen – which is the form in which glucose is stored in the body. Carbohydrates are obtained from food and are then broken down during digestion into simple sugars so that they can be absorbed through the mucous membrane of the digestive system into the blood and utilised by the body.

Lipids

Lipids include the fats, which are compounds of fatty acids and glycerol (Fig. 1.10) and are also made up of carbon, hydrogen and oxygen. Fatty acids are the main form in which fats are transported in the blood after the breakdown of lipids obtained from food. Although carbohydrates provide the most direct source of energy for the body, fats can also yield a large amount of energy. They are an important means of energy storage for the body, to be used when required. Other functions of lipids include insulation of the body itself and of nerves, and in the formation of cell membranes and synthesis of steroids.

Proteins

Proteins are built up from subunits called *amino acids* (Fig. 1.11). Proteins differ from carbohydrates and lipids in that they always contain nitrogen in addition to carbon, hydrogen and oxygen. They may also contain other elements such as sulphur, phosphorus and iodine. When two amino acids are joined together by a peptide link they form a dipeptide. The addition of more amino acids (a process called *polymerisation*) leads to the formation of a polypeptide. A protein consists of one or more polypeptide chains, which are

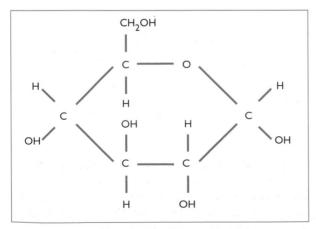

Fig. 1.9 Chemical structure of a simple carbohydrate – the sugar glucose.

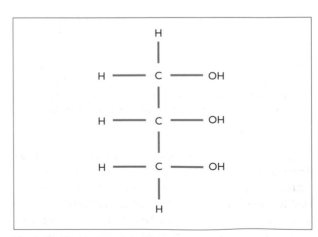

Fig. 1.10 Chemical structure of glycerol.

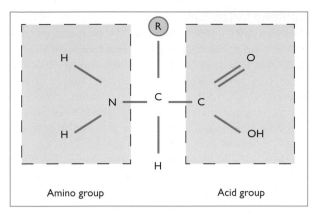

Fig. 1.11 General structure of an amino acid. The 'R' group varies from amino acid to amino acid.

then coiled and folded to give the specific structure of a particular protein (Fig. 1.12).

Proteins generally fall into one of two groups:

1. *Globular* – the functional proteins. These are associated with cellular chemical reactions and include hormones and enzymes
2. *Fibrous* – the structural proteins. These are insoluble and are part of the composition of various structures in the body. They include keratin, collagen and elastin.

By means of digestive enzymes the body breaks down the proteins acquired from the diet into their constituent amino acids, which can then be absorbed through the mucous membrane of the digestive system into the blood.

Chemical reactions in the body

Most of the chemical reactions that take place in the body require the presence of a functional protein compound called an *enzyme*. Enzymes are organic catalysts which speed up and control chemical reactions in the body. Enzymes are involved in the breakdown of food in the digestive system, but are also involved in the many metabolic processes that are carried out within cells.

> A chemical reaction that requires an input of energy is called an *anabolic* reaction. A chemical reaction that releases energy is a *catabolic* reaction. The sum of the energy use, i.e. the gain and loss, is the *total metabolism*.

All animals require energy and this is provided by raw materials obtained from food. This is then converted by the body into a form that it can use – adenosine triphosphate or ATP. Energy cannot be created or destroyed, it is just moved around or else changes its form, e.g. electrical energy can be converted to heat

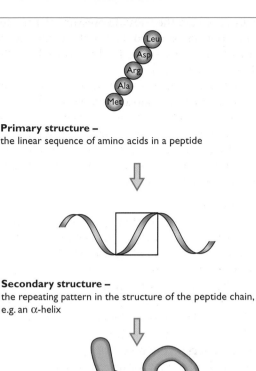

Primary structure –
the linear sequence of amino acids in a peptide

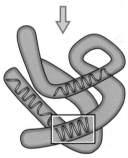

Secondary structure –
the repeating pattern in the structure of the peptide chain, e.g. an α-helix

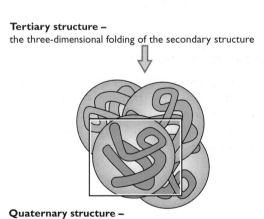

Tertiary structure –
the three-dimensional folding of the secondary structure

Quaternary structure –
the three-dimensional arrangement of more than one tertiary polypeptide

Fig. 1.12 The structure of a protein. It is not only the sequence of amino acids, but also the arrangement of the polypeptide chains, which determines the characteristics of a protein.

energy, or it can be stored as potential energy that is released when the compound in which the energy is stored is broken down. In the body of an animal, energy comes from the oxidation of glucose, i.e. a reaction involving oxygen and glucose.

🔑 KEY POINTS

- All living organisms can be classified into different orders, classes and families linked by certain common characteristics. These groups can be further divided into a genus and species which describes an individual type of organism.

- The body is made up of a number of systems, each of which has a specific function. These systems form the structural framework of the body or lie within one of three body cavities.

- Each system consists of a collection of tissues and organs which are comprised of the smallest units of the body – the cells.

- Cells can only be seen under the microscope and all have a basic structure with certain anatomical differences which adapt them to their specific function.

- Each structure within the cell plays a vital part in the normal function of the cell and therefore in the normal function of the body system.

- Cells grow and divide by means of mitosis. Each mitotic division results in the production of two identical daughter cells containing the diploid (or normal) number of chromosomes.

- The healthy body contains 60–70% water, distributed into two principal fluid compartments – the extracellular fluid (surrounding the cells) and the intracellular fluid (within the cells).

- Body fluids move between these compartments and this movement is controlled by the chemical constituents of the fluid and the physical processes of diffusion and osmosis.

- Body fluids contain inorganic and organic compounds. The structure and percentage of all of these is fundamental to the balance and normal function of the body. Within the body there are many systems involved in maintaining a state of equilibrium – this is known as homeostasis

Within the body individual cells are grouped together to forms tissues and organs. Thus:

- A *tissue* is a collection of cells and their products in which one type of cell predominates, e.g. epithelial tissue or muscle tissue.
- An *organ* is a collection of tissues forming a structure within an animal which is adapted to perform a specific purpose, e.g. liver, larynx, kidney.
- A *system* is a collection of organs and tissues which are related by function, e.g. respiratory system.

BODY TISSUES

Each tissue type consists of three main components:

1. Cells – one type forms the majority of the cells and gives the tissue type its name, e.g. muscle tissue consists mainly of muscle cells
2. Intercellular products – these are produced by the cells and lie in the spaces between them
3. Fluid – interstitial fluid flows through specialised channels running through the tissue.

There are four main types of tissue:

1. *Epithelial* – protects the body; may also be secretory and absorbent
2. *Connective* – binds the tissues together
3. *Muscle* – brings about movement
4. *Nervous* – conveys nerve impulses from one area to another and coordinates the response.

Epithelial tissue

Epithelial tissue or *epithelium* covers the surface of the body and the organs, cavities and tubes within it – it covers the internal and external surfaces of the body. Its main function is to protect delicate structures lying beneath it but in some areas the epithelium may be secretory, e.g. glands, or absorbent, e.g. in the small intestine. The epithelium lining structures such as the inside of the heart, blood vessels and lymph vessels is referred to as *endothelium*.

Epithelium may be described according to the number of layers of cells, i.e. its thickness:

- If an epithelium is one cell thick it is said to be *simple* (Fig. 2.1)
- If there is more than one layer it is said to be *stratified* or *compound* (Fig. 2.1).

The thickness of the epithelium reflects its ability to protect: the more layers of cells, the more protection is provided. The epithelium on the footpads consists of

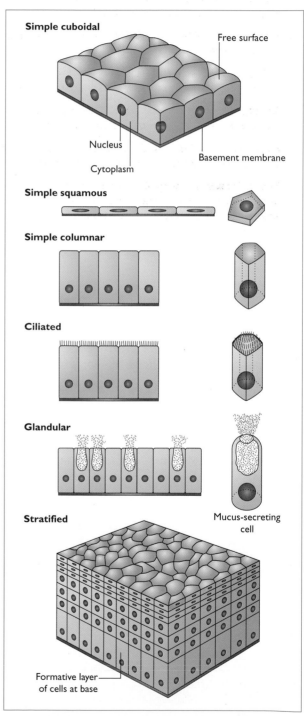

Fig. 2.1 The different types of epithelium found in the body.

many layers of cells providing protection when walking on rough surfaces, while the epithelium over the abdominal wall is only a few cells thick and additional protection is provided by fur. Further protection may be provided by the presence of the protein keratin. The epithelium is described as being a *keratinised stratified* epithelium and this type can be seen in claws and nails.

Epithelium may also be described according to the shape of the cells within it (Fig. 2.1). There are three basic shapes of epithelial cell:

1. *Squamous* cells – flattened in shape
2. *Cuboidal* cells – square or cube shaped
3. *Columnar* cells – column shaped (the height is greater than the width).

The full classification of the type of epithelium is based upon the shape of the cell and the number of layers present. There are a number of different types of epithelial tissue in the body, these include:

1. *Simple cuboidal epithelium* – this is the least specialised type of epithelium. It is one cell thick and the cells are cube shaped. Cuboidal epithelium lines many of the glands and their ducts. This type of epithelium has an absorptive or secretory function depending on its location in the body, e.g. lining the renal tubules.
2. *Simple squamous epithelium* – this type has flattened cells and is one layer thick. Simple squamous epithelium is thin and delicate and is found in areas of the body where the covering surface needs to be easily permeable to molecules such as oxygen, e.g. lining the blood vessels and the alveoli of the lungs.
3. *Simple columnar epithelium* – this has tall narrow cells and is one layer thick. Generally, simple columnar epithelium lines organs that have an absorptive function, e.g. the small and large intestines, or a secretory function, e.g. digestive glands.
4. *Ciliated epithelium* – this is a more specialised epithelium consisting of a single layer of columnar shaped cells (Fig. 2.1). The free surface of the cells has tiny hair like projections called *cilia* whose function is to 'waft' foreign particles along the epithelial surface and out of the body. Ciliated epithelium lines the upper respiratory tract, where it helps to trap solid particles that have been inhaled, preventing them from entering the more distal parts of the respiratory system. The uterine tubes are also lined with ciliated epithelium which helps to move the fertilised egg along the reproductive tract.
5. *Stratified epithelium* – this is composed of a number of layers of cells and is thicker and tougher than the other types of epithelium. It is found in areas that are subjected to wear and to friction and shearing forces, e.g. the epidermis of the skin (see page 151).
6. *Transitional epithelium* – a type of specialised stratified epithelium found lining parts of the urinary system, i.e. structures and tubes that are capable of considerable distension and variations in internal pressure and capacity, such as the bladder and ureters. The cells are able to change their shape according to circumstances and thus their appearance varies with the degree of distension of the structure.

Glands

Glandular tissue is a modification of epithelial tissue. The epithelium, in addition to its protective function, may also be a secretory membrane. Glands are either:

■ *Unicellular glands* – these have individual secretory cells are interspersed throughout the tissue. The most common type is the *goblet cell*, which secretes clear sticky mucus directly onto the membrane surface. The epithelium is known as a *mucous membrane*. Mucus traps particles, providing extra protection, and also lubricates the epithelial surface. Mucous membranes are found covering the oral cavity, lining the vagina and the trachea and in many other parts of the body.
■ *Multicellular glands* – these consist of many secretory cells folded to form more complex glands. They vary in shape and intricacy relating to their position and function in the body. Examples of some of the types of gland found in the body are shown in Figure 2.2.

Glands may be categorised as either:

■ *Exocrine glands* – these have a system of ducts through which their secretory products are transported directly to the site where they will be used
■ *Endocrine glands* – do not have a duct system (ductless glands) and their secretions, known as hormones, are carried by the blood to their target organ which may be some distance away (see Chapter 6).

Connective tissue

Connective tissue is responsible for supporting and holding all the organs and tissues of the body in place. It also provides the transport system within the body, carrying nutrients to the tissues and waste products away. Connective tissue consists of cells embedded in an extracellular *matrix* or *ground substance*. The properties of this ground substance depend on the type of connective tissue. There are many types of connective tissue which, in order of increasing density are:

Shape of gland		Type of gland	Location of gland
Tubular (single, straight)	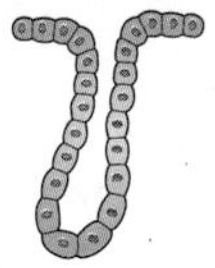	Simple tubular	Stomach, intestine
Tubular (coiled)	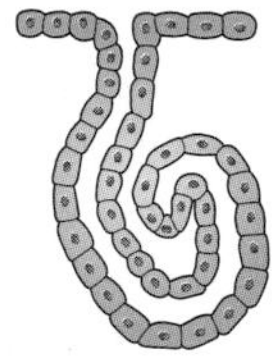	Simple coiled tubular	Sweat glands
Tubular (multiple)	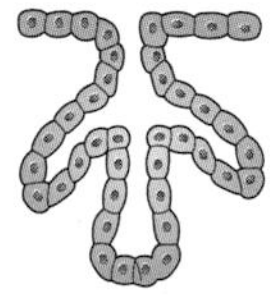	Simple branched tubular	Stomach, mouth, tongue, oesophagus
Alveolar (single)	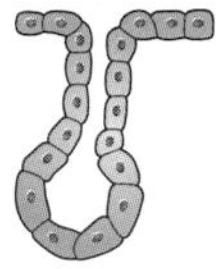	Simple alveolar	Sebaceous glands
Alveolar (multiple)	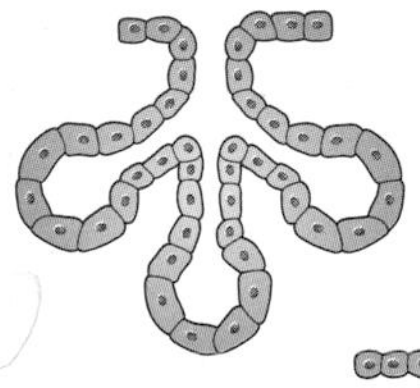	Branched alveolar (acinar)	Sebaceous glands
Tubular (multiple)	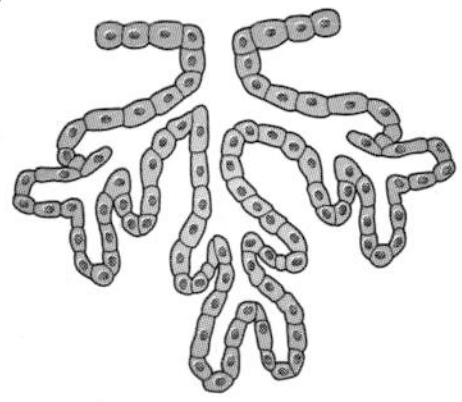	Compound tubular	Bulbourethral glands, mammary glands, kidney tubules, testes, mucous glands of the mouth
Alveolar (multiple)	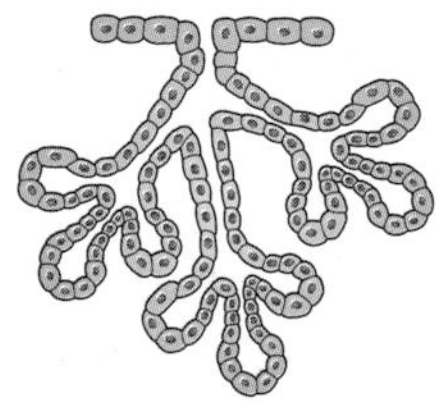	Compound alveolar (acinar)	Mammary glands
Some tubular; some alveolar	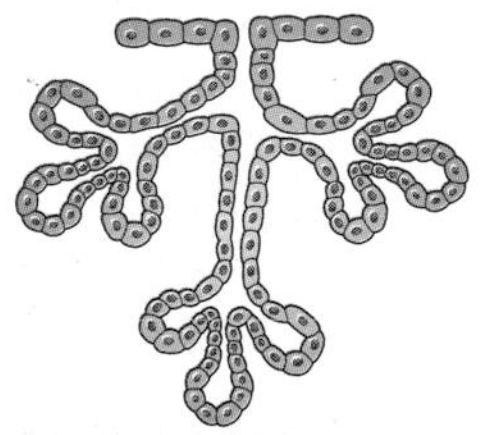	Compound tubuloalveolar	Salivary glands, pancreas, respiratory passages

Fig. 2.2 The different types of gland found in the body.

1. Blood
2. Haemopoietic tissue
3. Areolar tissue or loose connective tissue
4. Adipose or fatty tissue
5. Fibrous connective tissue or dense connective tissue
6. Cartilage
7. Bone.

Blood

Blood is a specialised connective tissue that circulates through the blood vessels to carry nutrients and oxygen to the cells, and waste products to the organs of excretion. It consists of a number of different types of blood cells within a fluid ground substance – the plasma. (This is covered in more detail in Ch. 7.)

Haemopoietic tissue

This jelly-like connective forms the bone marrow within the long bones and is responsible for the formation of the blood cells (see Chapter 7).

Areolar tissue (Fig. 2.3)

Areolar (meaning spaces) or loose connective tissue is the most widely distributed type of connective tissue and is found all over the body, e.g. beneath the skin, around blood vessels and nerves, between and connecting organs and between muscle bundles. The ground substance contains a loose weft work of two types of protein fibre: *collagen* fibres, with a high tensile strength secreted by the main cell type (the fibroblast) and *elastic* fibres, which enable the tissue to stretch and return to its former shape. Fat cells may be present in varying quantities depending on location and the degree of obesity of the animal. *Macrophages*, cells which are capable of phagocytosis, are also present.

Adipose tissue

Adipose tissue is similar to areolar tissue, but its matrix contains mainly fat filled cells, closely packed together, giving it the name fatty tissue. These fat cells act as an energy reserve and, in the dermis of the skin, the tissue insulates the body to reduce heat loss. In some areas such as around the kidney, adipose tissue provides a protective layer.

Dense connective tissue

Dense or fibrous connective tissue consists of densely packed collagen fibre bundles with relatively few fibroblasts and other cells in between them. The fibres may be arranged in two ways:

- Parallel arrangement – this is known as regular fibrous connective tissue, e.g. tendons, which are strong bands of fibrous tissue linking muscles to bone; and ligaments, which link bone to bone
- Irregularly interwoven fibres – this is seen in the dermis of the skin and in the capsules of joints, as well as in organs such as the testes and lymph nodes. Irregular dense connective tissue is often found in sheets and forms the basis of most fascias and aponeuroses.

Cartilage

Cartilage is a specialised connective tissue which is rigid but flexible and resilient and is able to bear weight (Fig. 2.4). It is composed of cells (known as *chondrocytes*) and fibres within a gel-like ground substance. Cartilage has no blood supply and its nutrition is supplied by the fibrous sheath or perichondrium that surrounds it.

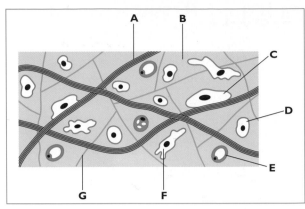

Fig. 2.3 Composition of areolar tissue. **A** Collagen fibres: flexible but very strong and resistant to stretching. **B** Ground substance: this contains the different fibres and cells of the tissue. **C** Fibroblast: long, flat cell which produces collagen and elastic fibres. **D** Mast cell: secretes an anticoagulant. **E** Fat cell: stores fat. **F** Macrophage: large cell capable of phagocytosis of foreign particles. **G** Elastic fibres: form a loose and stretchable network.

There are three types of cartilage:

1. *Hyaline cartilage* – this has a translucent, bluish-white appearance. The randomly arranged collagen fibres are not easily visible under the microscope as they have the same refractive index as that of the gel matrix. Hyaline cartilage is the most common type of cartilage in the body and forms the articular surfaces of joints, and provides support in the nose, larynx, trachea and bronchi. It also forms the skeleton of the embryo before it becomes ossified by the process known as *endochondral ossification*.
2. *Elastic cartilage* – this has chondrocytes within a matrix and numerous elastic fibres. Elastic cartilage occurs in places where support with flexibility is required, e.g. the external ear and epiglottis.
3. *Fibrocartilage* – this has a similar basic structure but has a higher proportion of collagen fibres giving it great strength, e.g. in the intervertebral discs, and in the menisci of the stifle joint. It also attaches the tendons and ligaments to bone.

Bone

Bone is a living tissue that is capable of remodelling and repairing itself when damaged. It is a specialised type of connective tissue, which provides the rigid supportive framework of the body and forms a system of levers for locomotion.

Bone consists of an extracellular matrix or ground substance that contains the protein osteonectin and collagen fibres. Together, these form *osteoid*, within

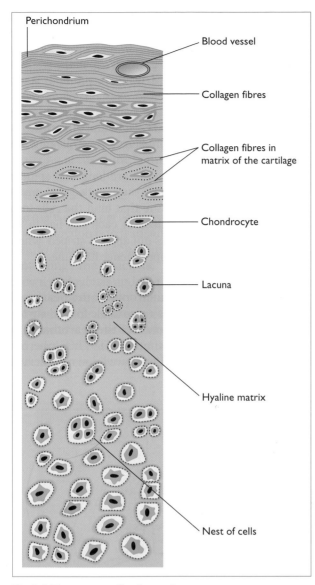

Fig. 2.4 The structure of hyaline cartilage.

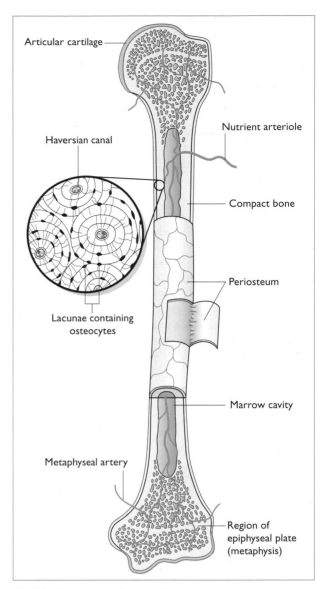

Fig. 2.5 The structure of compact bone.

which crystals of insoluble calcium phosphate are deposited as the bone tissue becomes calcified. Calcification gives bone its characteristic rigidity and hardness. As the ground substance becomes calcified the bone cells or *osteocytes* are trapped in spaces called *lacunae*. Running through the bone matrix are fine channels, called *Haversian canals*, which carry the blood vessels and nerves of the bone (Fig. 2.5). Each Haversian canal is surrounded by a series of concentric cylinders of matrix material called *lamellae* and the osteocytes within their lacunae. Each series of these cylinders, together with the canal, is called a *Haversian system* (Fig 2.5). A fibrous membrane, the *periosteum*, covers the outer surface of all types of bone.

There are two types of bone tissue:

1. *Compact bone* – this is solid and hard and is found in the outer layer or cortex of all types of bone. The Haversian systems of compact bone are densely packed together.
2. *Cancellous or spongy bone* – this consists of an internal meshwork of bony 'struts' or *trabeculae* with interconnected spaces between filled with red bone marrow. Cancellous bone is found in the ends of long bones, and in the core of short, irregular and flat bones.

Muscle tissue

Muscle tissue is responsible for organised movement in the body.

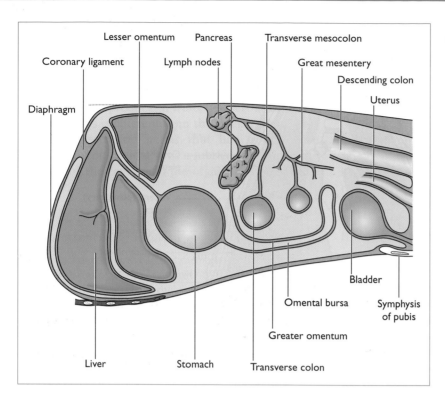

Fig. 2.12 Sagittal section through the abdominal cavity to show the reflections (folds) of the peritoneum.

Lesser omentum   Pancreas   Transverse mesocolon

Coronary ligament   Lymph nodes   Great mesentery

Descending colon

Uterus

Diaphragm

Bladder

Omental bursa   Symphysis of pubis

Greater omentum

Liver   Stomach   Transverse colon

🔑 KEY POINTS

■ The cells of the body are arranged into four basic tissue types: epithelial, connective, muscle and nervous tissue.

■ Epithelial tissue covers the outside of the body and lines all the body cavities and the structures within them. Its primary function is to protect but it in some areas it may also be absorbent or secretory. Secretory epithelial tissue forms glands.

■ Connective tissue is found in varying forms such as blood, fibrous connective tissue, cartilage and bone. Its main function is to connect and support the parts of the body, but it also carries nutrients to the tissues and conducts waste material away.

■ Muscle tissue brings about the movement of the body. It is found as striated muscle attached to the skeleton, smooth muscle within the internal organs of the body and cardiac muscle found only in the myocardium of the heart wall. Control of striated muscle is voluntary, while that of smooth and cardiac muscle is involuntary and brought about by branches of the autonomic nervous system.

■ Nervous tissue is found all over the body and its function is to conduct nerve impulses to and from parts of the body and the central nervous system.

■ The body is divided into three body cavities which contain the visceral systems. The thoracic and abdominal cavities are lined with a single layer of serous epithelial tissue which is named according to its location within the cavity.

THE SKELETAL SYSTEM

The skeletal system is the 'framework' upon which the body is built – it provides support, protection and enables the animal to move (Fig. 3.1). The joints are considered to be an integral part of the skeleton. The skeletal system is made of the specialised connective tissues bone and cartilage.

The functions of the skeletal system are:

1. *Support* – it acts as an internal 'scaffold' upon which the body is built
2. *Locomotion* – it provides attachment for muscles, which operate a system of levers, i.e. the bones, to bring about movement
3. *Protection* – it protects the underlying soft parts of the body, e.g. the brain is encased in the protective bony cranium of the skull
4. *Storage* – it acts as a store for the essential minerals calcium and phosphate
5. *Haemopoiesis* – haemopoietic tissue forming the bone marrow manufactures the blood cells.

BONE STRUCTURE AND FUNCTION

Bone shape

Bones can be categorised according to their shape:

- *Long bones* – these are typical of the limb bones, e.g. femur, humerus, and also include bones of the metacarpus/metatarsus and phalanges; long bones have a *shaft* containing a *medullary cavity* filled with bone marrow (Fig. 3.2).
- *Flat bones* – these have an outer layer of compact bone with a layer of cancellous or spongy bone inside, there is no medullary cavity, e.g. flat bones of the skull, scapula and ribs
- *Short bones* – these have an outer layer of compact bone with a core of cancellous bone and no medullary cavity, e.g. carpal and tarsal bones

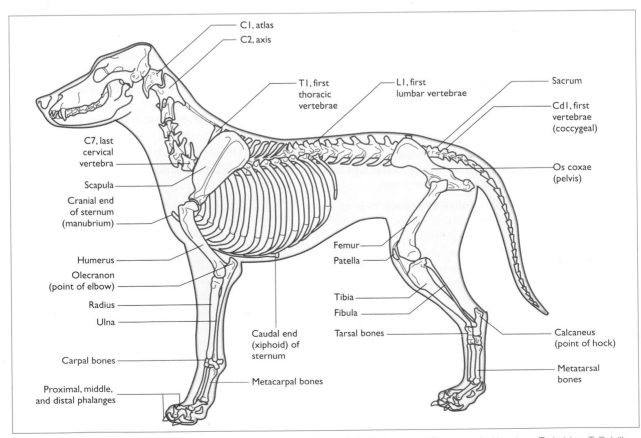

Fig. 3.1 The skeleton of the dog showing the major bones. (Reprinted from Clinical Anatomy and Physiology for Veterinary Technicians, T Colville and JM Bassett, p 102, Copyright 2002, with permission from Elsevier Science.)

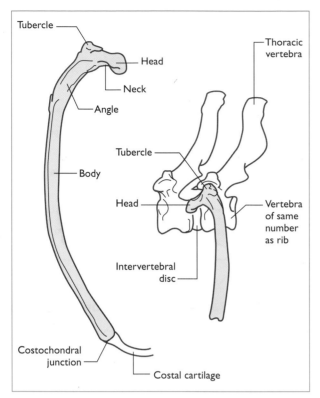

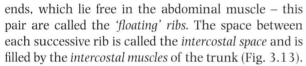

Fig. 3.12 Structure of the canine rib. **A** Caudal view. **B** Lateral view showing articulation with a thoracic vertebra. (Reprinted from Clinical Anatomy and Physiology for Veterinary Technicians, T Colville and JM Bassett, p 112, Copyright 2002, with permission from Elsevier Science.)

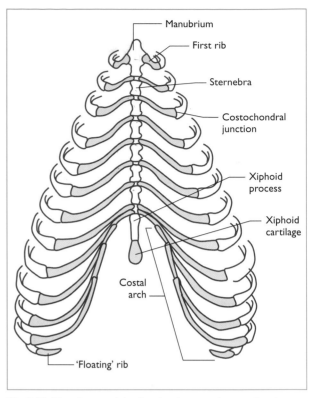

Fig. 3.13 The rib cage of the dog, showing sternal, asternal and 'floating' ribs. (Reprinted from Clinical Anatomy and Physiology for Veterinary Technicians, T Colville and JM Bassett, p 112, Copyright 2002, with permission from Elsevier Science.)

ends, which lie free in the abdominal muscle – this pair are called the *'floating' ribs*. The space between each successive rib is called the *intercostal space* and is filled by the *intercostal muscles* of the trunk (Fig. 3.13).

The sternum forms the floor of the thoracic cage (Fig. 3.13). and is composed of eight bones, the *sternebrae*, and the intersternebral cartilages. The most cranial sternebra is the *manubrium*, which projects in front of the first pair of ribs and forms part of the cranial thoracic inlet. Sternebrae 2–7 are short cylindrical bones. The last sternebra is longer and dorsoventrally flattened and is called the *xiphoid process*. Attached to the xiphoid process and projecting caudally is a flap of cartilage called the *xiphoid cartilage*. The linea alba attaches to this. Between each sternebra are cartilaginous discs called the *intersternebral cartilages*.

THE APPENDICULAR SKELETON

The appendicular skeleton is composed of the pectoral (or fore) limb and the pelvic (or hind) limb and the shoulder and pelvic girdles which attach these to the body. The forelimb has no bony connection to the trunk, only being attached by muscles. This absorbs

the 'shock' at the point when the limb takes the animal's weight in four legged animals or running quadrupeds. This differs from primates, which generally walk on their hind legs and so have evolved a pectoral girdle with a clavicle. However, the hindlimb does have a bony articulation in the pelvic girdle, which forms the platform for the muscles that provide the propulsive force as the animal is running.

Bones of the forelimb (Fig. 3.1)

The bones of the forelimb are:

- *Clavicle* – frequently absent in the dog. When present, it is just a remnant of bone that lies in the muscles cranial to the shoulder joint – it is described as being *vestigial*. The clavicle is normally present in the cat but does not articulate with other bones.
- *Scapula* – also called the shoulder blade (Fig. 3.14). It is a large flat bone found on the lateral surface of the trunk at the junction of the neck and ribs. It has a prominent ridge or *spine* running down the middle of its lateral surface. This divides the lateral surface into two regions: the *supraspinous fossa* and *infraspinous fossa*. On the distal end of the spine there is a bony projection called the *acromion*. At the

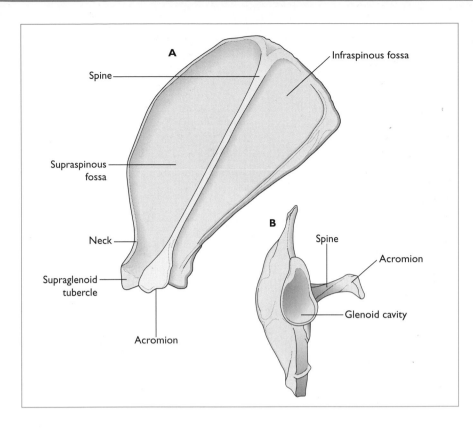

Fig. 3.14 The dog scapula.
A Lateral view. **B** Ventral view.

distal end of the scapula the bone narrows at the *neck* and there is a shallow articular socket, called the *glenoid cavity*, which forms the shoulder joint with the head of the humerus. The medial surface of the scapula is flat and comparatively smooth.

- *Humerus* – this a long bone forming the upper forelimb (Fig. 3.15). It articulates proximally with the scapula at the *shoulder joint*, and distally with the radius and ulna at the *elbow joint*. The proximal end of the humerus consists of a large rounded projection, the *head*. Cranial and lateral to the head there is a large prominence, called the *greater tubercle*. Another prominence, the *lesser tubercle*, lies medial to the head. Both of these are sites for attachment of the muscles that support the shoulder joint. Distal to the head is the *neck*, attached to the slightly twisted *shaft* of the bone. On the distal end of the humerus are the *medial* and *lateral epicondyles* between which is the *condyle*. Just proximal to this is a deep hollow called the *olecranon fossa*. This receives the anconeal process of the ulna. There is also a hole in the centre of the condyle called the *supratrochlear foramen*. N.B. There is no supratrochlear foramen in the cat.
- *Radius and ulna* – these are both long bones which lie side by side in the forearm (Fig. 3.16). At the proximal end of the ulna is a projection known as the *olecranon*, which forms the point of the elbow.

In front of this is a crescent shaped concavity called the *trochlear notch*, which articulates with the distal humerus. At the top of the trochlear notch is a beak-like projection called the *anconeal process*, which sits within the olecranon fossa of the humerus when the elbow is extended. Distally, the ulna narrows to a point called the *lateral styloid process*. The *radius* is a rod-like bone, shorter than the ulna (Fig. 3.16). At the proximal end is a depression, the *fovea capitis*, which articulates with the humerus. At the distal end of the radius there is a pointed projection called the *medial styloid process*.

APPLIED ANATOMY

The shaft of the humerus has a slight twist on it. If the humerus is broken, the resulting fracture is often in the form of a spiral.

APPLIED ANATOMY

Elbow dysplasia is a common condition of the heavier breeds of dogs, e.g. Newfoundland, St Bernard, Rottweiler, Basset. It encompasses a number of developmental conditions, such as an ununited anconeal process and detached olecranon process, which result in instability of the elbow joint, leading to osteoarthritis. The disease can be inherited and there is a BVA/KC scheme to identify affected individuals and to help breeders select the most suitable dogs for breeding.

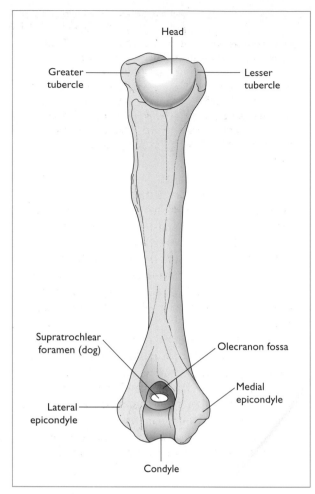

Fig. 3.15 The dog humerus. (Cats do not have a supratrochlear foramen.)

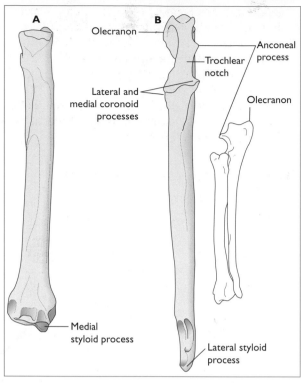

Fig. 3.16 **A** The dog radius. **B** The dog ulna (cranial and lateral views).

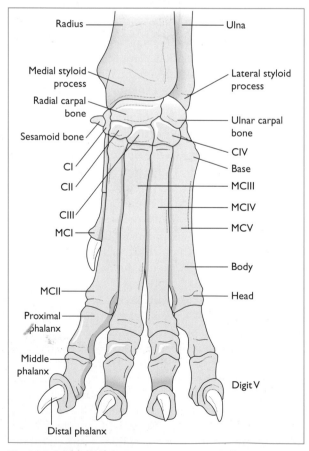

Fig. 3.17 Bones of the distal forelimb in the dog. CI, CII, etc. = carpal bones 1, 2, etc. MC = metacarpal bones. Metacarpal bone 1 is the dew claw.

■ *Carpus* – this is composed of seven short bones, the carpal bones, arranged in two rows. The proximal row has three bones, the most medial being the *radial carpal bone,* which articulates proximally with the radius. The *ulnar carpal bone* articulates proximally with the ulna. The *accessory carpal bone* lies on the lateral edge and projects caudally. Distally, the first row of carpal bones articulates with the second row of four carpal bones. The carpal bones also articulate with each other within the row.

■ *Metacarpus* – this is composed of five small long bones (Fig. 3.17). In the dog and cat the first metacarpal bone (I), i.e. the most medial, is much smaller than the other metacarpal bones (II–V), and is non-weight bearing. This forms part of the *dew claw.* The metacarpals articulate proximally with the distal row of carpal bones, and distally with the phalanges.

■ *Digits* – these are composed of the *phalanges,* which are long bones (Fig. 3.17). Each digit has three phalanges, except digit I – the dew claw – which has only two. The proximal phalanx articulates with a metacarpal bone. The middle phalanx articulates with the phalanx above and below it. The distal phalanx ends in the *ungual process* that forms part of the *claw*.

- There are pairs of small *sesamoid bones* behind the metacarpophalangeal joints and the distal joints between the phalangeal bones.

Bones of the hindlimb (Fig. 3.1)

The bones of the hindlimb are:

- *Pelvis* – this is the means by which the hindlimb connects to the body (Fig. 3.18). It consists of two hip bones or *ossa coxarum,* which join together at the *pubic symphysis.* They form a firm articulation with the sacrum at the *sacroiliac joint.* Each hip bone is formed from three bones – the *ischium, ilium* and *pubis* grouped around one very small bone called the *acetabular bone.* The largest of these bones is the ilium which has a broad cranial expansion called the *wing.* The ischium has a prominent caudal projection called the *ischial tuberosity.* The ilium, ischium and pubis meet each other at the *acetabulum,* which is the articular socket in which the head of the femur sits, forming the hip joint. The hip joint is a ball-and-socket joint.

- The head of the femur is held in place by a ligament known as the *teres* or *round ligament,* which attaches to a non-articular area within the joint cavity called the *acetabular fossa.* On either side of the pubic symphysis is a large hole called the *obturator foramen* which serves to reduce the weight of the pelvic girdle and to provide extra surface area for the attachment of muscles and ligaments.
- *Femur* – this is a long bone and forms the thigh (Fig. 3.19). On the proximal femur the articular head faces medially to articulate with the acetabulum of the pelvis. The head is joined to the shaft by a *neck.* Lateral to the head is a projection called the *greater trochanter* and on the medial side is another smaller projection called the *lesser trochanter.* Both of these are sites for muscle

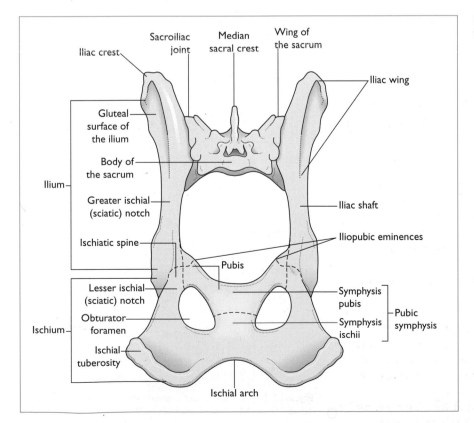

Fig. 3.18 Bones and bony features of the dog pelvis.

attachment. The femur has a strong shaft and on its distal extremity it has two caudally projecting *condyles:* the *medial condyle* and the *lateral condyle,* which articulate with the tibia at the *stifle joint.* The *patella* runs between these condyles in the *trochlea groove.*

- The *patella* is a sesamoid bone found within the tendon of insertion of the *quadriceps femoris* muscle, which is the main extensor of the stifle (see Ch. 4 and (Fig. 3.23). Two more sesamoid bones, called the *fabellae* are found behind the stifle in the origin of the *gastrocnemius* muscle. They articulate with the condyles of the femur.
- *Tibia and fibula* – these long bones form the lower leg (Fig. 3.20). The tibia and fibula lie parallel to each other, the more medial bone, the tibia, being the much larger of the two. The tibia is expanded proximally where it articulates with the femur. On the dorsal surface there is a prominence called the *tibial crest* for attachment of the quadriceps femoris muscle. Distally, the tibia has a prominent protrusion, the *medial malleolus,* which can be palpated on the medial aspect of the hock. The fibula is a thin long bone lying laterally to the tibia. It ends in a bony point called the *lateral malleolus.*
- *Tarsus* – this is formed from seven short bones, the *tarsal bones,* arranged in three rows (Fig. 3.21).

APPLIED ANATOMY

In some small breeds of dog, e.g. Yorkshire Terrier, the patella may slip out of place causing extreme pain and difficulty in extending the stifle joint. This is an inherited condition and is due to malpositioning of the tibial crest or too shallow a trochlea groove on the distal end of the femur.

The two bones forming the proximal row, the *talus* and *calcaneus,* articulate with the distal end of the tibia and fibula at the hock joint (see Fig. 3.23, p. 43). The talus, or tibial tarsal bone, is the most medial and has a proximal trochlea, which is shaped to fit the end of the tibia. The calcaneus, or fibular tarsal bone, is positioned laterally and has a large caudal projection known as the *tuber calcis,* which forms the 'point' of the hock.

- *Metatarsus and digits* – these closely resemble the pattern of the metacarpus and digits in the forepaw. The metatarsus is composed of four metatarsal bones, although some breeds possess five, having a small metatarsal I or hind dew claw.

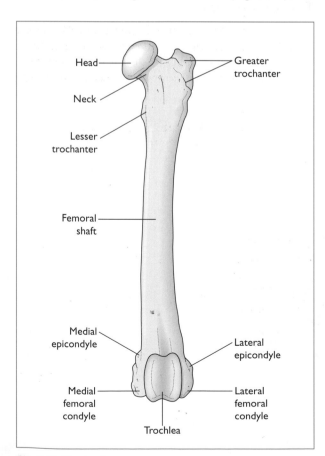

Fig. 3.19 The dog femur.

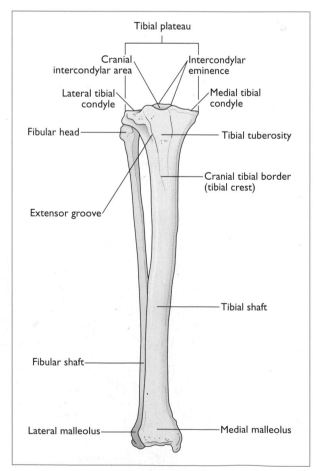

Fig. 3.20 The dog tibia and fibula.

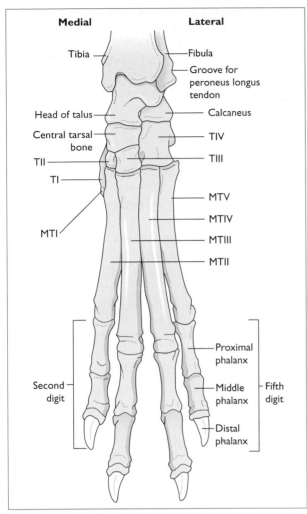

Fig. 3.21 The dog tarsus or hindpaw. TI, TII, etc. = tarsal bones 1, 2, etc. MT = metatarsal bones.

Splanchnic skeleton

This is composed of the splanchnic bones. A splanchnic bone is a bone that develops in soft tissue and is unattached to the rest of the skeleton. The only example of a splanchnic bone in the dog and cat is the bone of the penis, the *os penis*. The urethra lies in the *urethral groove* on the ventral surface of the os penis in the dog. In the cat the urethral groove is on the dorsal surface of the os penis, due to the different orientation of the penis (see Ch. 11).

The cow has a splanchnic bone in its heart, called the *os cordis*, while the bird has splanchnic bones forming a rim around the eye to provide strength to the large eyeball (see Ch. 13).

JOINTS

When one bone connects to another they form an articulation, also known as an *arthrosis* or *joint*. Joints allow variable degrees of movement and can be categorised into one of three groups:

1. Fibrous joints
2. Cartilaginous joints
3. Synovial joints.

Fibrous joints

Fibrous joints are immovable joints and the bones forming them are united by dense fibrous connective tissue, e.g. in the skull, fibrous joints unite the majority of the component bones and are called *sutures*. The

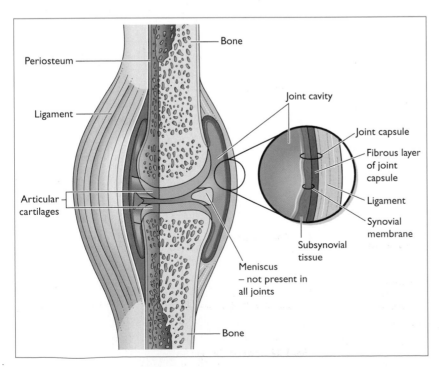

Fig. 3.22 Structure of a typical synovial joint.

teeth are attached to the bony sockets in the jaw bone by fibrous joints.

Fibrous joints are also classed as *synarthroses*, i.e. a type of joint that permits little or no movement. Some cartilaginous joints also fall into this category.

Cartilaginous joints

Cartilaginous joints allow limited movement or no movement at all and are united by cartilage, e.g. the *pubic symphysis* connecting the two hip bones, and the *mandibular symphysis* joining the two halves of the mandible. Both these joints are also classed as *synarthroses*.

Some cartilaginous joint may also be classed as *amphiarthroses*, which allow some degree of movement between the bones, e.g. between the bodies of the vertebrae, allowing for limited flexibility of the spinal column.

Synovial joints

Synovial joints or *diarthroses* allow a wide range of movement. In synovial joints, the bones are separated by a space filled with synovial fluid known as the *joint cavity* (Fig. 3.22). A joint capsule surrounds the whole joint; the outer layer consists of fibrous tissue, which serves as protection, and the joint cavity is lined by the *synovial membrane*, which secretes *synovial fluid*. This lubricates the joint and provides nutrition for the hyaline articular cartilage covering the ends of the bone. Synovial fluid is a straw coloured viscous fluid that may be present in quite large quantities in large joints, especially in animals that have a lot of exercise.

Some synovial joints may have additional stabilisation from thickened *ligaments* within the fibres of the joint capsule. These are most commonly found on either side of the joint, called *collateral ligaments*. However, other synovial joints have stabilising ligaments attached to the articulating bones within the joint – these are known as *intracapsular ligaments* and examples include the cruciate ligaments within the stifle joint (Fig. 3.23).

A few synovial joints possess one or more intra-articular fibrocartilaginous *discs* or *menisci* within the joint cavity. These are found in the stifle joint – it has two crescent shaped menisci – and in the temporomandibular joint between the mandible and the skull. These structures help to increase the range of movement of the joint and act as 'shock absorbers,' reducing wear and tear.

Synovial joints allow considerable freedom of movement between the articulating bones, the extent of which depends upon the type of synovial joint. The movement allowed by a synovial joint may be in a single plane only, or in multiple planes.

The range of movements that are possible in synovial joints are:

- *Flexion/extension* – these are antagonistic movements of a joint.
  - Flexion *reduces* the angle between two bones, i.e. bends the limb
  - Extension *increases* the angle between two bones, i.e. straightens the limb
- *Abduction/adduction* – these movements affect the whole limb:
  - Abduction (meaning to 'take away') moves a body part *away* from the median plane or axis, e.g. moving the leg out sideways
  - Adduction moves a body part back *towards* the central line or axis of the body, e.g. moving the leg back to standing position
- *Rotation* – the moving body part 'twists' on its own axis, i.e. it rotates either inwardly or outwardly
- *Circumduction* – the movement of an extremity, i.e. one end of a bone, in a circular pattern
- *Gliding/sliding* – the articular surfaces of the joint slide over one another
- *Protraction* – the animal moves its limb cranially, i.e. advances the limb forward, as when walking
- *Retraction* – the animal moves the limb back towards the body.

Synovial joints can be further classified into subcategories based upon the types of movement that they allow (Table 3.1).

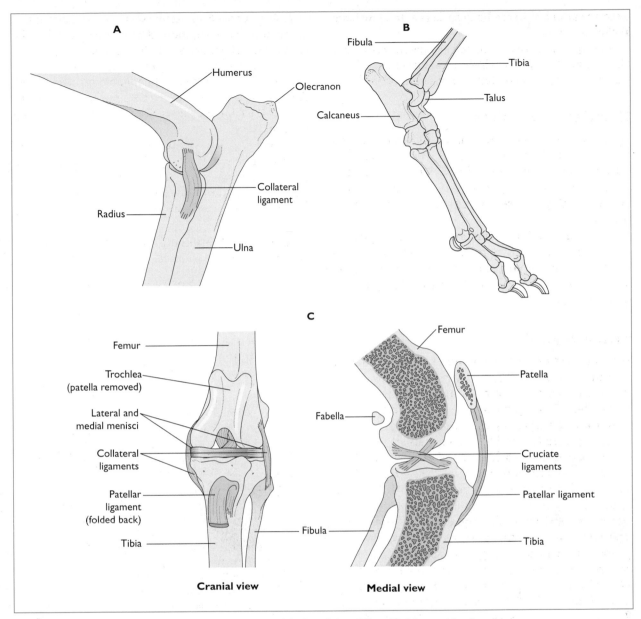

A

Humerus

Olecranon

Radius

Collateral ligament

Ulna

B

Fibula

Tibia

Talus

Calcaneus

C

Femur

Trochlea (patella removed)

Lateral and medial menisci

Collateral ligaments

Patellar ligament (folded back)

Tibia

Femur

Patella

Fabella

Cruciate ligaments

Patellar ligament

Fibula

Tibia

Cranial view

Medial view

Fig. 3.23 **A** The elbow joint, lateral view. **B** The tarsus or hock joint, lateral view. **C** The stifle joint, cranial and medial views.

Table 3.1 Properties of different synovial joint types.

Type of synovial joint	Description	Example of joint
Plane/gliding	Allows sliding of one bony surface over the other	Joints between the rows of carpal and tarsal bones
Hinge	Allows movement in one plane only, i.e. flexion and extension	Elbow; stifle
Pivot	Consists of a peg sitting within a ring; allows rotation	Atlanto-axial joint (between C1 and C2)
Condylar	Consists of a convex surface (condyles) that sits in a corresponding concave surface; allows movement in two planes (flexion, extension and over extension)	Hock or (tarsus)
Ball and socket	Consists of a rounded end or ball, sitting within a socket or cup; allows a great range of movement	Hip; shoulder

🔑 KEY POINTS

■ The skeletal system provides a supporting framework for the body, a firm base to which the muscles of locomotion are attached, and protects the softer tissues enclosed within the framework.

■ The skeleton can be considered to be made up of three parts:
1. Axial skeleton, forming the central axis of the animal and comprising the skull, vertebral column and the rib cage
2. Appendicular skeleton, comprising the fore and hind limbs and the limb girdles which attach them to the body
3. Splanchnic skeleton, which in the dog and cat consists only of the os penis found within the soft tissues of the penis.

■ Each part of the skeleton consists of many bones, each of which plays an important part in the function of the skeletal system.

■ Bones are covered in 'lumps, bumps and holes'. Each has a specific descriptive name and a function which contributes to movement, i.e. muscle attachment, or to maintaining the health of the tissue, i.e. blood or nerve supply.

■ Bones are linked together by means of joints.

■ Joints can be classified according to the type of tissue from which they are made, e.g. fibrous, cartilaginous or synovial joints, or according to the type of movements they allow, e.g. hinge or gliding joints.

THE MUSCULAR SYSTEM

The muscular system includes all the skeletal or striated muscles within the body. Striated muscle is that tissue attached to the skeleton and which is under voluntary or conscious control (for microscopic structure see Ch.2).

MUSCLE STRUCTURE AND FUNCTION

Contraction

Muscle is stimulated to contract when it receives a nerve impulse from the central nervous system. Each striated muscle fibre is composed of myofibrils made of thin *actin* filaments and thick *myosin* filaments. These fibres overlap in such a way that under the microscope muscle has the appearance of alternating light and dark bands or striations. These bands are separated into units called *sarcomeres*, which are the units of contraction.

During contraction, the actin and myosin filaments slide over one another and cross-bridges form between the heads of the myosin filaments and the heads of the actin filaments. The cross-bridges swing through an arc, pulling the thin filaments past the thick ones, and the sarcomere shortens. Once this movement is completed the cross-bridge detaches itself from the thin filament and reattaches itself further away – in other words, the cross-bridges between the myosin and actin filaments act as a ratchet mechanism, thus shortening the muscle (Fig. 4.1). This process requires energy input, which is provided by ATP molecules; calcium ions are also essential to the process of muscle contraction.

The nerve that stimulates the muscle to contract enters the muscle and then splits up into many fibres to innervate the bundles of muscle fibres. The number of muscle fibres supplied by one nerve fibre will vary depending on the type of movement for which the

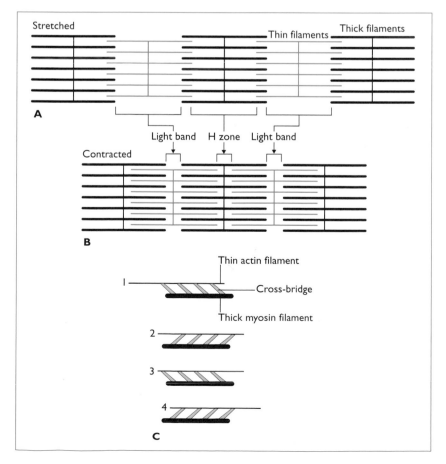

Fig. 4.1 The 'ratchet mechanism' involving actin and myosin within striated muscle fibres. **A** Muscle before contraction (shortening). **B** When the muscle shortens, the thick and thin filaments slide in between one another. The dark bands remain the same width in the shortened (contracted) muscle, but the light bands and 'H zones' get narrower. **C** Close up view of the 'ratchet mechanism', showing cross-bridges between the thin actin and thick myosin filaments.

- *Pectineus* – this muscle runs from the pubis to the distal
  ACTION – adducts the limb
- *Sartorius* – inserts on the cranial border of the tibia with the gracilis muscle
  ACTION – adducts the limb
- *Gracilis* – forms the caudal half of the medial surface of the thigh
  ACTION – adducts the limb

Muscles of the lower hindlimb

These muscles act mainly on the hock joint (Fig. 4.13). They include:

- *Gastrocnemius* – this muscle originates from the caudal aspect of the femur and inserts on the calcaneus of the hock. The tendons of this muscle contain two small sesamoid bones or fabellae that articulate with the caudal aspect of the stifle joint
  ACTION – extends the hock and flexes stifle

- *Achilles tendon* – this is the large strong tendon that runs down the back of the leg to the point of the hock. It includes the tendons of insertion of the gastrocnemius, biceps femoris and semitendinosus, all of which insert on the calcaneus, and also of the superficial digital flexor muscle, which continues over the point of the hock and down to its insertion on the digits. There is a bursa at the point of insertion on the calcaneus.

Muscles of the hock and digits

As is seen in the forelimb, there are a number of muscles responsible for flexing and extending the hock and the digits:

- *Anterior tibialis* – runs from the proximal end of the tibia to the tarsus
  ACTION – flexes the hock and rotates the paw medially
- *Three digital extensors* – run in front of the hock and foot
- *Two digital flexors* – run behind the foot. The *superficial digital flexor* runs from the femur to the phalanges and is one of the components of the Achilles tendon.

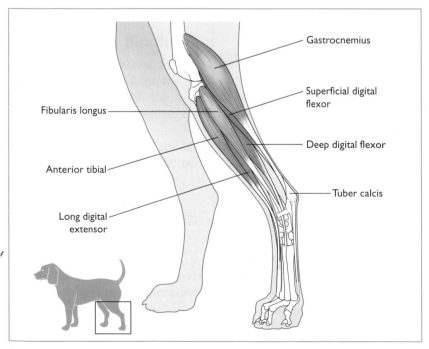

Fig. 4.13 Muscles of the lower left hindlimb.

🔑 KEY POINTS

■ The muscular system comprises striated or skeletal muscle, i.e. muscle which is attached to the skeleton and brings about movement of a region.

■ Each striated muscle fibre is filled with myofibrils made of two contractile proteins, actin and myosin. At the cellular level, muscle contraction results from the formation of cross-bridges between the actin and myosin molecules.

■ Muscle fibres are stimulated to contract by nerve impulses carried by nerve fibres. The number of muscle fibres supplied by a single nerve fibre is called a motor unit. In muscles which perform accurate and delicate movements, a nerve fibre will supply a few muscle fibres, but in muscles which perform less accurate movements a nerve fibre will supply many muscle fibres.

■ Muscle tissue is always under a degree of tension, known as muscle tone. The tone increases when an animal is alert or frightened and decreases when it is relaxed or asleep.

■ All muscles consist of a central belly and, at the point of attachment to a bone, an origin (often called the head), and an insertion.

■ Skeletal muscles may be either:
– Extrinsic, i.e. attached from one major structure, such as the trunk, to another structure, such as a limb. These muscles bring about movement of the *whole* limb in relation to other body parts
– Intrinsic, i.e. attached at both ends within the one structure, such as a limb. These muscles bring about movement *within* the individual limb, e.g. bending an elbow.

■ Each area has a range of specialised muscles designed to bring about the specific types of movement necessary for the animal's normal function.

Table 5.2 The autonomic nervous system.

	Sympathetic system	Parasympathetic system
Origin of nerve fibres	Vertebrae T1 to L4 or L5	Cranial nerves III, VII, IX, X; vertebrae S1, S2
Preganglionic nerve fibres	Short; each nerve leads to a ganglion containing cell bodies and lying close under the vertebral column; there is a chain of ganglia – the sympathetic chain – one on each side of the vertebral column	Long; ganglia lie close to the organ they supply; there is no chain of ganglia
Postganglionic nerve fibres	Long; lead away from the sympathetic chain and travel towards the organ it supplies – usually follow the path of blood vessels	Short; fibres run a short distance from the ganglion to the organ
Areas supplied	Viscera in thorax, abdomen and pelvis; also supply sweat glands, blood vessels and piloerector muscles associated with hair follicles. Most ganglia are paired, but three are unpaired: 1. Coeliac – supplies stomach, small intestine, pancreas, large intestine and adrenal medulla 2. Cranial (superior) mesenteric – supplies large intestine 3. Caudal (inferior) mesenteric – supplies bladder and genitals	Structures in the head including the eye and salivary glands; vagus (X) supplies the heart, lungs, stomach, small intestine, pancreas and large intestine
Transmitter substances:		
A. Within the system, i.e. between cell body and dendron	Acetyl choline	Acetyl choline
B. At the terminal synapses, i.e. between the axon and the effector organ	Noradrenaline	Acetyl choline
General effect	Prepares the body for 'fear, flight, fight'; heart and respiratory rates are increased, blood vessels to skeletal muscle are dilated, blood glucose levels rise, piloerector muscles to the hairs contract so hackles are raised, GI tract activity decreases	Animal is more relaxed; heart rate is slowed, respiratory bronchioles constrict, GI tract activity increases – digestive juices and salivary secretion increases, peristalsis increases

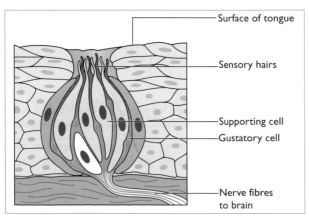

Fig. 5.12 Cross-section through a taste bud.

to the nasal cavities and dorsal to the mouth. The dog and the cat are predatory species and their eyes point forwards (Fig. 5.13). This provides a wide area of binocular or 3D vision, enabling them to pinpoint the position of their prey accurately. Prey species such as the rabbit or the mouse have prominent eyes set on the sides of the head. These provide a wide area of monocular or 2D vision which enables the animal to see the predator but not to fix its position – this does not matter, the important factor is that the predator is nearby and that the prey animal runs.

Each eye consists of three main parts: the eyeball, the extrinsic muscles and the eyelids.

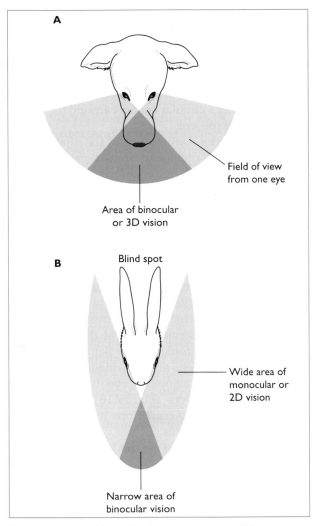

Fig. 5.13 Fields of vision. **A** Predator animal, e.g. dog. **B** Prey animal, e.g. rabbit.

The eyeball (Fig. 5.14)

The eyeball is a globe-shaped structure made of three layers:

1. The *sclera*
2. The *uvea*
3. The *retina*.

Sclera

The *sclera* forms the fibrous outer covering of the eye, in conjunction with the *cornea*.

- *Cornea* – covering ⅙ of the eyeball, the cornea forms the transparent anterior part of the eye and bulges slightly outwards from the orbit. It has a poor blood supply but is well supplied with sensory nerve fibres. The outer surface is covered in a layer of squamous epithelium, the *conjunctiva*. The cornea is the first part of the eye to be hit by rays of light and is involved in focusing these on to the retina.
- *Sclera* – covering ⅚ of the eyeball, the sclera is dull white in colour. It consists of dense fibrous connective tissue and elastic fibres into which the extrinsic muscles insert. Its function is to protect the delicate internal structures of the eye and to maintain the eye shape.

The junction between the cornea and sclera is known as the *limbus*. This is the drainage point for the aqueous humour of the anterior chamber of the eye.

Uvea

The *uvea*, a vascular pigmented layer, is firmly attached to the sclera at the exit of the optic nerve, but

Fig. 5.14 Structure of the canine and feline eye.

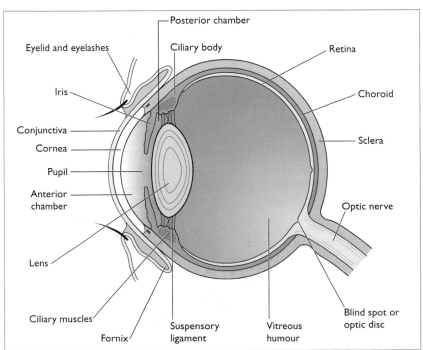

this part of the pituitary gland are secreted by the hypothalamus and only stored here. They are:

- *Antidiuretic hormone* (ADH) – also called vasopressin. This hormone alters the permeability of the collecting ducts of the kidney to water. It is secreted in response to the changing volume of extracellular fluid (ECF) and helps maintain homeostasis.
- *Oxytocin* – this has two effects:
  - It acts on the mammary glands during late pregnancy and causes the milk to be released or 'let down' in response to suckling by the neonate
  - At the end of gestation, oxytocin causes the contraction of the smooth muscle of the uterus, resulting in parturition and delivery of the fetuses.

Thyroid glands

These lie in the midline on the ventral aspect of the first few rings of the trachea (Fig 6.1). They are controlled by thyroid or thyrotrophic stimulating hormone (TSH) from the anterior pituitary gland, and secrete three hormones:

- *Thyroxin* (or T_4) and *tri-iodothyronine* (or T_3) – have a similar effect. Tri-iodothyronine contains a high proportion of the trace element iodine – a lack of iodine in the diet can have a dramatic effect. Both hormones affect the uptake of oxygen by all the cells in the body and are essential for normal growth.

Undersecretion – *hypothyroidism* – is more common in dogs. In young animals, hypothyroidism causes *dwarfism* (stunted growth). In older animals, the condition is known as *myxoedema:* the dog becomes fat and sluggish, alopecic, the skin feels cold and clammy and the heart rate slows – all due to a reduced metabolic rate.
Oversecretion – *hyperthyroidism* – is more common in old cats. The affected animal is thin, active, often aggressive, has a good appetite and a fast heart rate – all due to a raised metabolic rate.

- *Calcitonin* – lowers the levels of blood calcium by decreasing the rate of bone resorption. When levels of blood calcium are high, e.g. if a calcium rich diet is eaten, calcium is deposited in the bone and acts as a reservoir for later use (Fig. 6.2). Calcitonin has an opposite effect to parathormone but is of less importance.

Parathyroid glands

These glands lie on either side of the thyroid gland and secrete the hormone *parathormone* (Fig. 6.1). Secretion is dependent on the levels of calcium in the blood – if levels are low, calcium is resorbed from the bones and absorption of calcium from the intestine is increased (Fig. 6.2).

Oversecretion *(hyperparathyroidism)* occurs in:

- *Primary hyperparathyroidism* – due to neoplasia of the parathyroid glands. This causes bone resorption, bone weakness and pathological fractures.
- *Secondary hyperparathyroidism* – as seen in chronic renal failure. The calcium:phosphate ratio in the blood is altered by impaired kidney function. This leads to increased output of parathormone and consequently increased resorption of bone in an effort to maintain blood calcium levels. There is preferential resorption from the mandible and maxilla, producing a condition known as 'rubber jaw' – the jaw becomes pliable and fragile and the teeth may fall out.
- *Nutritional hyperparathyroidism* – results from feeding low calcium diets, e.g. all meat diet. Parathormone is produced in an attempt to raise the blood calcium levels by bone resorption.

Pancreas

The pancreas is a pinkish lobulated gland lying in the loop of the duodenum in the abdominal cavity (Fig. 6.1).

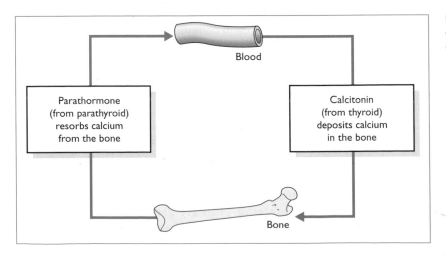

Fig. 6.2 Control of blood calcium levels by Calcitonin and parathormone.

It has an exocrine part and an endocrine part and is described as being a *mixed gland.* The exocrine secretions enter the duodenum via the pancreatic duct (see Chapter 9). The endocrine secretions are produced by discrete areas of tissue within the exocrine tissue, known as the *islets of Langerhans.*

The islets of Langerhans secrete three hormones, each from a different type of cell:

1. *Insulin* (from the β cells) – secreted in response to high blood glucose levels. Insulin lowers blood glucose levels by:
   - Increasing the uptake of glucose into the cells, where it is metabolised to provide energy
   - Storing excess glucose as glycogen in the liver. Conversion of glucose to glycogen occurs by a process known as *glycogenesis* (Fig. 6.3).

> Lack of insulin leads to a condition known as *diabetes mellitus,* in which the animal suffers from hyperglycaemia and glucosuria (the presence of glucose in the urine). If left untreated, the condition may progress to a stage where the body uses its protein and fat stores as a source of energy. Daily insulin injections and dietary control are necessary to control the condition.

2. *Glucagon* (from the α cells) – secreted in response to low blood glucose levels. Glucagon raises blood glucose levels by breaking down the glycogen stores in the liver. Conversion of glycogen to glucose occurs by a process known as *glycogenolysis* (Fig. 6.3).
3. *Somatostatin* (from the δ cells) – this is mildly inhibitory to the secretions of insulin and glucagon and prevents wild fluctuations in blood glucose levels. It also decreases gut motility and the secretion of digestive juices, which serve to reduce the efficiency of the digestive and absorptive processes.

Ovaries

At the onset of sexual maturity, the ovaries become capable of secreting two hormones:

1. *Oestrogen* – produced by the walls of the developing *ovarian follicles.* Development of germ cells in the ovary into ripe follicles is the result of the secretion of FSH from the anterior pituitary gland. Oestrogen causes the behaviour associated with the oestrous cycle and prepares the reproductive tract and external genitalia for mating (see Ch. 11). Oestrogen also exerts negative feedback on the anterior pituitary gland, preventing further secretion of FSH and further follicular development (Fig. 6.4).
2. *Progesterone* – secreted by the *corpus luteum,* which develops from the remaining follicular tissue after the follicle has ovulated. The corpus luteum develops as a result of the production of LH from the anterior pituitary gland. Progesterone prepares the reproductive tract for pregnancy and maintains the pregnancy (see Ch. 11). During pregnancy, progesterone exerts negative feedback on the hypothalamus and prevents secretion of *gonadotrophin releasing hormone* and so prevents further oestrous cycles until parturition occurs. It also causes development of the mammary glands during pregnancy (Fig. 6.4).

In the later stages of pregnancy, the corpus luteum also secretes a hormone known as *relaxin.* This causes the sacroiliac and other ligaments around the birth canal to soften and relax in preparation for parturition.

Testes

At the start of sexual maturity, the testes begin to secrete two hormones:

1. *Testosterone* – produced by the *interstitial cells* or *cells of Leydig* in response to the secretion of ICSH

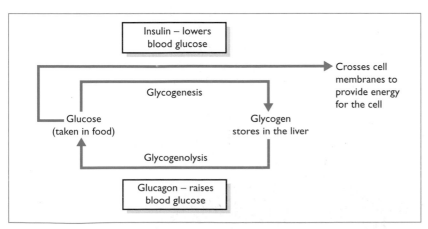

Fig. 6.3 Control of blood glucose levels.

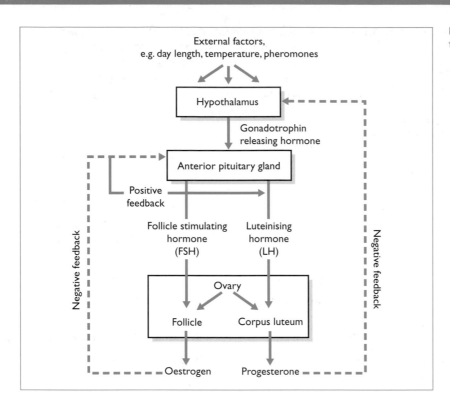

Fig. 6.4 Inter-relationships between the female reproductive hormones.

from the anterior pituitary gland. Testosterone is responsible for:
- The development of male characteristics such as muscle development, size or jowls on the face of a tomcat
- Male behaviour patterns, e.g. aggression, territorial behaviour, courtship displays and mating behaviour
- Development of spermatozoa.

2. *Oestrogen* – produced by the *Sertoli cells* in the seminiferous tubules of the testes.

Adrenal glands

There is a pair of adrenal glands, one lying close to the cranial pole of each kidney (Fig. 6.1). Each gland has an outer *cortex* and an inner *medulla*. There is no connection between the two parts and they can be considered as two separate glands.

Adrenal cortex

The hormones produced are known as *steroids* and have a similar structure based on lipid. There are three groups, each one being secreted by a different layer:

1. *Glucocorticoids* – secretion is regulated by ACTH from the anterior pituitary gland. The hormones are known as *corticosteroids;* the most important are *cortisol* and *corticosterone.* In the normal animal they are present in low levels but increase in response to stress. They have two main actions:
- They increase blood glucose levels by reducing glucose uptake by the cells, increasing the conversion of amino acids to glucose in the liver (a process known as *gluconeogenesis*) and mobilising fatty acids from the adipose tissue ready for conversion to glucose.
- When present in large quantities, they depress the inflammatory reaction, which delays healing and repair. This property is used therapeutically to reduce swelling and inflammation.

Oversecretion of glucocorticoids, or *hyperadrenocorticalism,* leads to symptoms of Cushing's disease. These include polydipsia, polyuria, polyphagia and bilateral symmetrical alopecia.

2. *Mineralocorticoids* – the most important is *aldosterone.* This acts on the distal convoluted tubule of the kidney where it regulates acid/base balance of the plasma and ECF by excretion of H^+ ions and also controls the excretion of Na^+ and K^+ ions.

3. *Adrenal sex hormones* – both male and female animals produce all types of sex hormones. They are secreted in insignificant quantities, but may be the reason why some animals show a certain level of sexual behaviour despite being neutered.

Adrenal medulla

This produces two hormones with similar actions *Adrenaline* (epinephrine) and *noradrenaline* (norepinephrine). These hormones prepare the body for emergency action, known as the 'fear, flight, fight' syndrome and are controlled by the sympathetic nervous system. Their actions are to:

1. Raise blood glucose levels by the breakdown of glycogen stored in the liver – *glycogenolysis.* This increases the body's energy levels.
2. Increase the heart rate and the rate and depth of respiration – this increases the amount of oxygen reaching the tissues.
3. Dilate the blood vessels of the skeletal muscles – this enables the supply of glucose and oxygen to reach the areas where it is needed.
4. Decrease the activity of the gastrointestinal tract and the bladder – in an emergency their functions are less important.

KEY POINTS

- The endocrine system is part of the regulatory system of the body and works in conjunction with the nervous system. The nervous system produces an immediate response while the endocrine system produces a slower but longer lasting effect.

- Endocrine glands secrete hormones which are carried by the blood to specific target organs.

- Each target organ responds only to a particular hormone or to a group of hormones and is unaffected by other hormones.

- Hormonal secretion is controlled by different mechanisms, e.g. levels of a chemical in the blood, or by a feedback loop.

- Each hormone has a specific effect and many interrelate with other hormones to create a complex network which acts to maintain the body in a state of equilibrium.

The blood vascular system is made up of four parts:

1. *Blood* – a fluid connective tissue which transports oxygen and nutrients around the body and collects waste products produced by the tissues.
2. The *heart* – a hollow muscular four-chambered organ responsible for pumping blood around the body.
3. The *circulatory system* – a network of arteries, veins and capillaries in which the blood flows around the body.
4. The *lymphatic system* – a network of lymphatic vessels which transports lymph or excess tissue fluid around the body and is responsible for returning it to the circulation.

BLOOD

Blood is a highly specialised fluid connective tissue (see Ch. 2), consisting of several types of cell suspended in a liquid medium called *plasma*. Blood makes up about 7% of the total body weight and has a pH of about 7.4. (7.35–7.45).

Functions

Blood has many functions within the body but they can be broadly divided into two groups: transport and regulation.

Transport

- *Gases in solution* – blood carries oxygenated blood from the lungs and delivers the oxygen to the tissues where it is used. It then collects deoxygenated blood containing carbon dioxide produced by the tissues during their metabolic processes, and carries it back to the lungs, where the carbon dioxide is exchanged for oxygen in the inspired air.
- *Nutrients* – blood transports nutrients, e.g. amino acids, fatty acids and glucose which result from the process of digestion, from the digestive system to the liver and to the tissues where they are needed.
- *Waste products* – blood collects the waste products resulting from metabolism in the tissues and transports them to the kidney and liver where they are excreted from the body.
- *Hormones and enzymes* – blood transports enzymes and hormones from the endocrine glands to their target tissues.

Regulation

Blood plays a vital role in homeostasis by regulating:

- *Volume and constituents of the body fluids* – blood carries water in the form of plasma to the tissues and is responsible for maintaining the osmotic balance of the fluids and the cells. The presence of plasma proteins, particularly albumin in the blood, controls the flow of fluid between the fluid compartments and is responsible for maintaining blood volume and blood pressure.
- *Body temperature* – blood conducts heat around the body to the body surface where if necessary it is lost by peripheral vasodilation.
- *Acid/base balance* – blood maintains a constant internal pH in the body by the presence of buffers, e.g. bicarbonate, which are able to absorb H^+ ions when the blood is acid (low pH) and give out H^+ ions when the blood is alkaline (high pH). In this way, all the processes of the body are able to function effectively.
- *Defence against infection* – blood helps to prevent infections through the action of the white blood cells, which are part of the body's immune system. It also carries antibodies and antitoxins produced by the immune system around the body.
- *Blood clotting* – the clotting mechanism prevents excessive blood loss from wounds and other injuries and prevents the entry of infection.

Composition of blood

Blood is a red fluid which is carried by the blood vessels of the circulatory system. It is composed of a fluid part, the *plasma,* and a solid part, the *blood cells* (Fig. 7.1). Plasma forms part of extracellular fluid (ECF) (see Ch. 1). Each constituent of the blood plays a specific part in the overall function of blood.

Plasma

Plasma is the liquid part of the blood which separates out when a blood sample is spun in a centrifuge. The main constituent is water (about 90%) in which are a number of dissolved substances being transported from one part of the body to another. These include carbon dioxide in solution, nutrients such as amino acids, glucose and fatty acids, waste materials such as urea, hormones, enzymes, antibodies and antigens.

In addition to these, plasma contains:

- *Mineral salts* – the main mineral salts found in extracellular fluid are sodium and chloride, but potassium, calcium, magnesium and bicarbonate are also present. The functions of these mineral salts include maintaining osmotic balance and maintaining pH by acting as buffers. Calcium has a number of essential roles in the body, e.g. in blood clotting, muscle contraction and nerve function.

■ *Plasma proteins* – these help to maintain the osmotic pressure of the blood because they are too large to pass out of the circulation. This has the effect of retaining fluid in the blood by osmosis, i.e. it prevents too much water from 'leaking' out into the extracellular spaces. If this did occur then the volume of the blood would decrease and the blood pressure would fall with serious consequences. The most important proteins are:

  – *Albumin:* helps to maintain the osmotic concentration of the blood, i.e. holds the water in the blood
  – *Fibrinogen* and *prothrombin:* involved in the clotting mechanism of the blood
  – *Immunoglobulins:* these are the antibodies produced by the immune system of the body.

Albumin, fibrinogen and prothrombin are produced by the liver, but the immunoglobulins are produced by the cells of the immune system.

Blood cells

The blood cells (Fig. 7.1) make up the solid component of blood and can be divided into three types:

1. *Erythrocytes* – the red blood cells
2. *Leucocytes* – the white blood cells
3. *Thrombocytes* – the platelets, which are cell fragments.

Before studying the different types of blood cell it is useful to understand a number of terms.

Haemopoiesis – the formation of all types of blood cell

Erythropoiesis – the formation of red blood cells or erythrocytes

Lymphoid tissue – found in the lymph nodes and spleen and produces agranular leucocytes, i.e. lymphocytes and monocytes

Myeloid tissue – found in the red bone marrow and is responsible for the formation of erythrocytes and granular leucocytes, i.e. neutrophils, eosinophils and basophils

Serum – plasma minus the clotting factors fibrinogen and prothrombin. It can be obtained by allowing a blood sample to clot naturally.

Erythrocytes (or red blood cells)

Erythrocytes are the most numerous blood cell – there are about 6–8 million per cubic mL of blood (Fig. 7.2). Their function is to transport oxygen and a small proportion of carbon dioxide around the body (most carbon dioxide is carried in solution in the plasma).

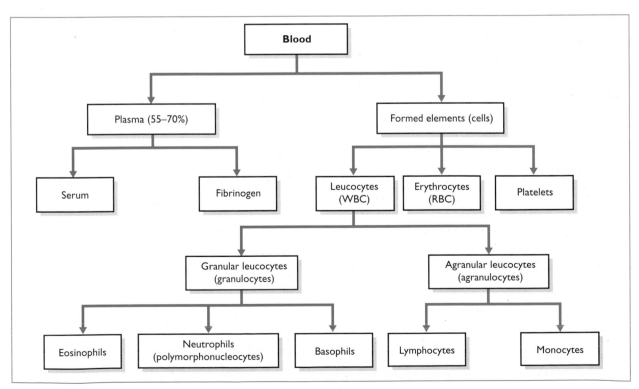

Fig. 7.1 The composition of blood.

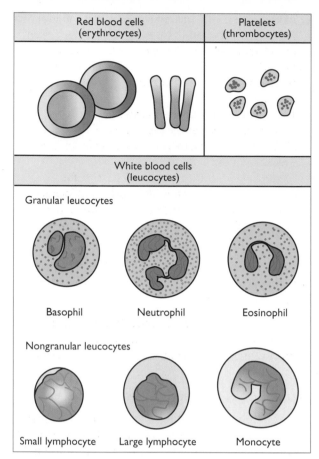

Red blood cells (erythrocytes)	Platelets (thrombocytes)

White blood cells (leucocytes)

Granular leucocytes

Basophil   Neutrophil   Eosinophil

Nongranular leucocytes

Small lymphocyte   Large lymphocyte   Monocyte

Fig. 7.2 The cellular components of blood. (Reprinted from Clinical Anatomy and Physiology for Veterinary Technicians, T Colville and JM Bassett, p 197, Copyright 2002, with permission from Elsevier Science.)

Mature erythrocytes are biconcave circular discs of about 7 μm in diameter. Erythrocytes contain a red pigment called *haemoglobin*, which is a complex protein containing iron. They are the only cells in the body without a nucleus, which allows a greater amount of haemoglobin to be packed into a relatively small cell. Erythrocytes are surrounded by a thin flexible cell membrane which enables them to squeeze through capillaries. Their shape and thin cell membrane gives them a large surface area for gaseous exchange and allows oxygen to diffuse across into the cell where it combines with the haemoglobin to form *oxyhaemoglobin*.

Erythrocytes are formed from undifferentiated *stem cells* within the bone marrow by a process known as *erythropoiesis*. The stem cells change into *erythroblasts*, which have a nucleus. The cell begins to acquire haemoglobin and its nucleus shrinks – it is now known as a *normoblast*. As the cell develops further it becomes a *reticulocyte*, at which point the nucleus consists only of fine threads in the cytoplasm known as *Howell-Joly bodies*. Eventually, the nucleus disappears and the mature erythrocyte is released into the circulation. This process takes 4–7 days.

If there is a shortage of erythrocytes, e.g. acute haemorrhage or iron-deficiency anaemia, reticulocytes are also released into the circulation to help make up the deficit. These can be seen on a blood smear stained with methylene blue which is a specific stain for reticulocytes.

A circulating erythrocyte has a lifespan of about 120 days, after which it is destroyed in the spleen or lymph nodes. The iron from the haemoglobin is recycled back to the bone marrow and the remainder is converted by the liver into the bile pigment *bilirubin* and excreted in bile.

The production of red blood cells is controlled by a hormone called *erythropoietin* (see Ch. 6) which is released by cells in the kidney in response to low oxygen levels in the tissues. Erythropoietin stimulates the stem cells in the bone marrow to produce more erythrocytes.

Leucocytes (or white blood cells)

Leucocytes are much less numerous than red blood cells and the cells contain nuclei. Leucocytes can be classified as either *granulocytes* or *agranulocytes* depending upon whether or not they have visible granules in their cytoplasm when stained and viewed under a microscope (Fig. 7.2). The function of leucocytes is to defend the body against infection.

Granulocytes This type of leucocyte is produced within the bone marrow and they make up approximately 70% of all leucocytes. They have granules within their cytoplasm and have a segmented or lobed nucleus which can vary in shape. They are referred to as polymorphonucleocytes or PMNs (meaning many-shaped nuclei). They can be further classified according to the type of stain they take up, i.e. neutral, basic or acidic. There are three types of granulocytes:

1. *Neutrophils* – take up neutral dyes and the granules stain purple (Fig. 7.2). Immature neutrophils have a nucleus that looks like a curved band and are known as *band cells*. Neutrophils are the most abundant of the leucocytes, forming about 90% of all granulocytes. They are able to move through the endothelial lining of the blood vessels into the surrounding tissues and engulf invading bacteria and cell debris by phagocytosis, thus helping to fight disease. A *neutrophilia* or raised numbers of neutrophils indicates the presence of an infective process while a *neutropaenia* or lack of white cells may be characteristic of certain viral infections.
2. *Eosinophils* – these take up acidic dye and the granules in their cytoplasm stain red (Fig. 7.2). They are involved in the regulation of the allergic and inflammatory processes and they secrete enzymes which inactivate histamine. Eosinophils play a major role in controlling parasitic

infestation. An *eosinophilia* or raised numbers of eosinophils occurs in response to parasitic infestation.

3. *Basophils* – these take up basic or alkaline dyes and the granules in the cytoplasm stain blue (Fig. 7.2). Basophils secrete *histamine,* which increases inflammation, and *heparin,* which is a natural anticoagulant preventing the formation of unnecessary blood clots. Basophils are present in very small numbers in normal blood.

Agranulocytes   Agranulocytes have a clear cytoplasm. There are two types:

1. *Lymphocytes* – this is the second most common type of white blood cell, forming 80% of all agranulocytes (Fig. 7.2). Lymphocytes are the main cell type of the immune system and are formed in lymphoid tissue although they originate from stem cells in the bone marrow. Lymphocytes are responsible for the specific immune response, and there are two different types: the *B-lymphocytes* which produce antibodies and are involved in humoral immunity, and the *T-lymphocytes* which are involved in the cellular immune response.
2. *Monocytes* – these have a horse shoe shaped nucleus and are the largest of the leucocytes, though they are only present in small numbers (Fig. 7.2). They are *phagocytic* cells and when they migrate to the tissues they mature and become known as *macrophages.*

Thrombocytes

Thrombocytes, or *platelets*, are cell fragments formed in the bone marrow from large cells called *megakaryocytes*. They are small discs with no nuclei and are present in the blood in large quantities. Platelets are involved in blood clotting.

Blood clotting

The ability to form a blood clot is one of the most important defence mechanisms in the body. It means that injured blood vessels can be sealed and excessive blood loss can be prevented. Blood clotting is essential for wound healing and also prevents the entry of pathogenic microorganisms into the wound. The formation of a blood clot is complicated and involves a number of different chemical factors in the blood. It is described as a *cascade mechanism* because one step leads on to another in a similar way to a cascade of water.

To simplify the process we will only consider the main steps. When a blood vessel or a tissue is damaged the following happens:

1. Platelets stick to the damaged blood vessel and each other to form a seal. The platelets release an enzyme called *thromboplastin.*
2. In the presence of thromboplastin and calcium ions, the plasma protein *prothrombin* is converted to the active enzyme *thrombin* (vitamin K is essential to the blood clotting mechanism and is required for the manufacture of prothrombin in the liver).
3. Thrombin then converts the soluble plasma protein *fibrinogen* into a meshwork of insoluble fibres called *fibrin.* The presence of calcium is an essential factor.
4. The fibrin fibres form a network across the damaged area that traps blood cells and forms a *clot.* This seals the vessel in what is often called a 'scab' and further blood loss from the wound is prevented.

The normal *clotting time* in a healthy animal is 3–5 minutes but it may be affected by a number of factors. It may be reduced by:

- Surface contact with materials that will act as foundation for the clot, e.g. gauze swabs
- Raising the environmental temperature – keeping the animal in a warm kennel.

Clotting time may be increased by:

- Lack of vitamin K, which is needed by the liver to form prothrombin in the blood (seen in warfarin poisoning, which interferes with levels of vitamin K)
- Liver disease – the liver manufactures the plasma proteins involved in clotting
- Genetic factors, e.g. haemophilia, which affects the availability of some clotting factors
- Systemic diseases such as anthrax, canine infectious hepatitis and viral haemorrhagic disease all cause subcutaneous haemorrhages due to interference with blood clotting
- Thrombocytopaenia – lack of platelets may be seen in some forms of leukaemia
- Lack of blood calcium – this feature is used in the lab to prevent blood samples clotting. Chemicals such as EDTA (ethylene diamine tetra-acetic acid), citrate and oxalate all combine with calcium in the blood and prevent it being involved in the clotting process.

The body has its own natural anticoagulant, called *heparin,* which prevents unwanted clots forming in the blood vessels and organs. If part of a clot, referred to as an *embolus,* detaches, it may be carried around the body and block any of the vital blood vessels, killing the animal.

THE HEART

The heart is a muscular organ that contracts rhythmically, pumping the blood through the blood vessels and around the body (Fig. 7.3). The heart is enclosed

THE LYMPHATIC SYSTEM

The lymphatic system is part of the circulatory system of the body and is responsible for returning the excess tissue fluid that has leaked out of the capillaries to the circulating blood. The fluid within the system is called *lymph* and is similar to plasma but without the larger plasma proteins. However, lymph contains more lymphocytes than are present in the blood. The lymphatic system is composed of both lymphatic vessels and lymphoid tissue, which are found in all regions of the body with a few exceptions such as the central nervous system and bone marrow.

The functions of the lymphatic system are:

- To return excess tissue fluid that has leaked out of the capillaries to the circulating blood
- To remove bacteria and other foreign particles from the lymph in specialised filtering stations known as lymph nodes
- To produce lymphocytes which produce antibodies; the lymphatic system may also be considered as part of the immune system
- To transport the products of fat digestion and the fat-soluble vitamins from the lacteals of the intestinal villi to the circulation.

The lymphatic system consists of the following parts:

- Lymphatic capillaries
- Lymphatic vessels
- Lymphatic ducts
- Lymph nodes
- Lymphatic tissues.

Lymphatic capillaries

Excess tissue fluid is collected up by the smallest of the lymphatic vessels, the *lymphatic capillaries*. These are thin-walled delicate tubes, which form networks within the tissues. In the villi of the small intestine the lymph capillaries are called *lacteals* and are responsible for collecting up the products of fat digestion (see Ch. 9).

Lymphatic vessels

The lymphatic capillaries merge to form the larger *lymphatic vessels*, which have a similar structure to veins and possess numerous closely spaced valves. Lymph flow is mainly passive and relies on the contraction of the surrounding muscles to move the lymph along. The valves prevent backflow and pooling of lymph in the vessels.

Lymphatic ducts (Fig. 7.7)

The lymphatic vessels enter the larger *lymphatic ducts* which drain lymph into blood vessels leading to the heart and so return it to the circulation. The major lymphatic ducts are:

1. The *right lymphatic duct* – this is the smaller of the two major ducts and drains lymph from the right side of the head, neck and thorax, and right forelimb. It empties into the right side of the heart via either the right jugular vein or cranial vena cava.
2. The *thoracic duct* – this is the main lymphatic duct and collects blood from the rest of the body. It arises in the abdomen, where it is called the *cisterna chyli*, and receives lymph from the abdomen, pelvis and hindlimbs. As it passes through the aortic hiatus of the diaphragm and enters the thorax, it becomes known as the *thoracic duct* and receives lymph from the left side of the upper body and left forelimb. The thoracic duct empties into either the jugular vein or cranial vena cava, near the heart.
3. There is also a pair of *tracheal ducts* that drain the head and neck and empty either into the thoracic duct or one of the large veins near the heart.

Lymph nodes (Fig. 7.8)

The lymph nodes are masses of lymphoid tissue situated at intervals along the lymphatic vessels (Fig. 7.7). They are bean shaped and have an indented region, called the *hilus*, where the lymph vessels leave the

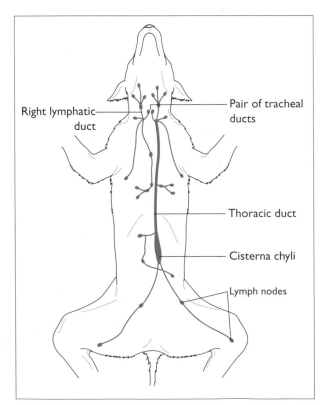

Fig. 7.7 Location of the lymphatic vessels and lymph nodes.

Right lymphatic duct

Pair of tracheal ducts

Thoracic duct

Cisterna chyli

Lymph nodes

node. A number of *afferent lymphatic vessels* carry lymph to each lymph node and enter the node on its convex surface. The lymph leaves the node at the hilus in the single *efferent vessel.*

Each node is surrounded by a fibrous connective tissue *capsule.* Inside, a network of tissue, called *trabeculae,* extends from the capsule and provides support for the entire node. The tissue of the node is divided into cortical and medullary regions. The cortex contains the germinal centres or *lymph nodules* that produce the *lymphocytes,* which play an important part in the immune system. The medulla is comprised of a reticular framework containing many phagocytic cells. Lymph flows through *spaces* or *sinuses* within the tissue of the node.

All lymph must pass through at least one lymph node before being returned to the circulation. Each node acts as a mechanical filter, trapping particles such as bacteria within the meshwork of tissue. The particles are then destroyed by phagocytic cells. Lymph nodes are distributed throughout the body and range in size. They can become enlarged during infection and are an indication of a disease process in the drainage region. In a generalised infection or disease all the lymph nodes may be enlarged.

Some lymph nodes are superficial and can be palpated (Fig. 7.9). These include:

- *Submandibular nodes* – 2–5 nodes in a group, lying at the edge of the angle of the jaw
- *Parotid node* – lies just caudal to the temporomandibular joint of the jaw
- *Superficial cervical nodes* also called the *prescapular nodes* – two on each side lying just in front of the shoulder joint, at the base of the neck on the cranial edge of the scapula
- *Superficial inguinal nodes* – two nodes on each side lying in the groin, between the thigh and the abdominal wall, dorsal to the mammary gland or penis
- *Popliteal node* – lies within the tissue of the gastrocnemius muscle, caudal to the stifle joint.

Lymphatic tissues

These include organs which contain lymphoid tissue and play an important part in the body's defence system.

Spleen

This is the largest of the lymphoid organs. The spleen is found within the greater omentum closely attached to the greater curvature of the stomach. It is a dark red haemopoietic organ which is not essential for life. The spleen has a number of functions:

1. Storage of blood – it acts as a reservoir for red blood cells and platelets
2. Destruction of worn out red blood cells – the phagocytic cells engulf and destroy the erythrocytes, and preserve their iron content for re-use in haemoglobin synthesis

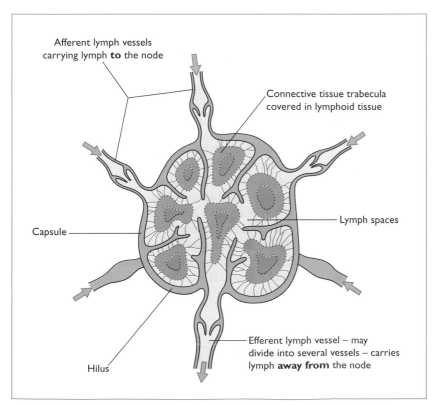

Fig. 7.8 Structure of a lymph node.

after swallowing the epiglottis falls forward, opening the glottis and thus allowing the passage of air to resume.

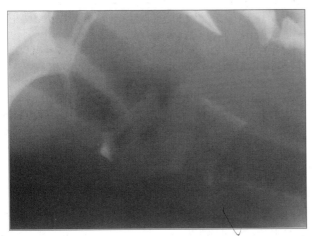

Fig. 8.3 Lateral view of dog's laryngeal area, showing the cartilages of the hyoid apparatus as they appear on X-ray.

APPLIED ANATOMY

Laryngeal paralysis is a condition seen in older dogs, often of larger breeds, e.g. Labradors. The vocal folds hang within the lumen of the larynx and are unable to move out of the flow of air. This results in interference with the passage of air down the larynx and trachea which could result in asphyxiation during exercise. It also causes a constant 'roaring' sound as the dog breathes.

Within the larynx is a pair of *vocal ligaments*. The mucous membrane covering the inner surface of the vocal ligaments forms the *vocal folds*, which project bilaterally into the lumen of the larynx. When air moves past the vocal folds they vibrate and sound is produced. These sounds can be modified by factors such as the size of the glottis and the tension of the vocal folds, resulting in a characteristic range of sounds, e.g. growling, barking, purring.

Trachea

From the larynx, air enters the *trachea*. This is a permanently open tube attached to the caudal border of the laryngeal cartilages (Fig. 8.4). It lies on the ventral aspect of the neck, i.e. below the oesophagus and slightly to the right of it, and extends the length of the neck, passing through the cranial thoracic inlet. In the thoracic cavity it enters the mediastinum and terminates at a *bifurcation* above the heart.

The lumen of the trachea is kept open by a series of C-shaped rings of hyaline cartilage. These prevent the trachea from collapsing when the thoracic pressure falls and the incomplete rings allow food boluses to pass down the oesophagus unimpeded by the tracheal cartilages. The structure of the trachea is flexible to allow movement of the head and neck. The cartilage rings are connected by fibrous tissue and smooth muscle fibres.

The trachea is lined with *ciliated mucous epithelium*. The surface layer of mucus traps any foreign particles

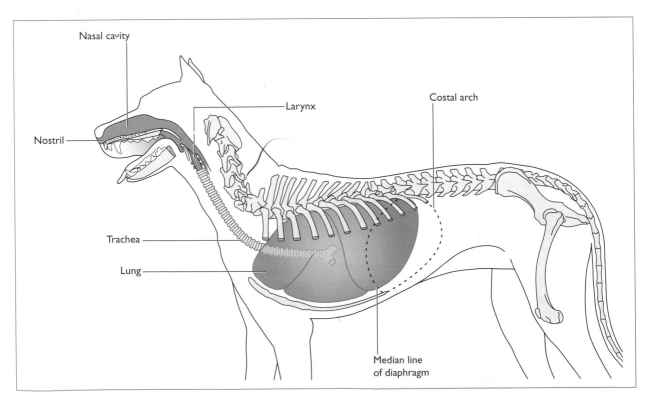

Fig. 8.4 Diagram illustrating the trachea and lung positions.

and the cilia 'sweep' the particles and mucus upwards to the pharynx, where they are spat out or swallowed. In some cases, such as in a dusty or smoky atmosphere, the production of mucus may increase. This mucus irritates the tracheal lining and causes the animal to cough. The *coughing reflex* serves to expel substances such as excess mucus and dust particles from the respiratory tract, preventing them from entering the lungs and is part of the animal's primary defence system.

Bronchi and bronchioles

The trachea divides (or bifurcates) into the right and left *bronchi* (sing. *bronchus*), entering each of the lungs respectively. As they enter the lung tissue the bronchi divide into smaller and smaller branches, like a tree. This arrangement is therefore known as the *bronchial tree.*

The bronchi are supported by complete rings of cartilage, but as the branches become smaller the cartilaginous support gradually diminishes, and then disappears completely, at which point the passages are called *bronchioles*. The bronchioles continue to branch into smaller passages throughout the lungs. Finally, the smallest diameter branches are known as the *alveolar ducts* and lead to the *alveoli.*

The walls of the bronchi and bronchioles contain smooth muscle, which is under the control of the autonomic nervous system. The respiratory passages are able to dilate to enable a greater volume of air to reach the lungs, e.g. during exercise, or constrict to their original size during 'normal' breathing.

Alveoli

The alveolar ducts end as the *alveolar sacs,* which resemble bunches of grapes. Each alveolar sac consists of a large number of alveoli, which are small, thin-walled sacs surrounded by capillary networks (Fig. 8.5). The epithelial lining of the alveolus is called the *pulmonary membrane,* and is very thin to allow gaseous exchange with the blood to take place. Oxygen in the inspired air diffuses across the pulmonary membrane of the alveolus into the blood within the capillaries of the pulmonary circulation. Simultaneously, it is exchanged for carbon dioxide in

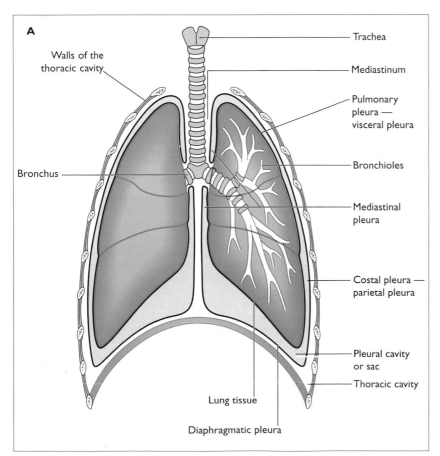

Fig. 8.5 The lungs within the thoracic cavity. **A** The pleural membranes. **B** (overleaf) The terminal air passages. (Part **B** reprinted from Clinical Anatomy and Physiology for Veterinary Technicians, T Colville and JM Bassett, p 227, Copyright 2002, with permission from Elsevier Science.)

A

Walls of the thoracic cavity

Bronchus

Trachea

Mediastinum

Pulmonary pleura — visceral pleura

Bronchioles

Mediastinal pleura

Costal pleura — parietal pleura

Pleural cavity or sac

Thoracic cavity

Lung tissue

Diaphragmatic pleura

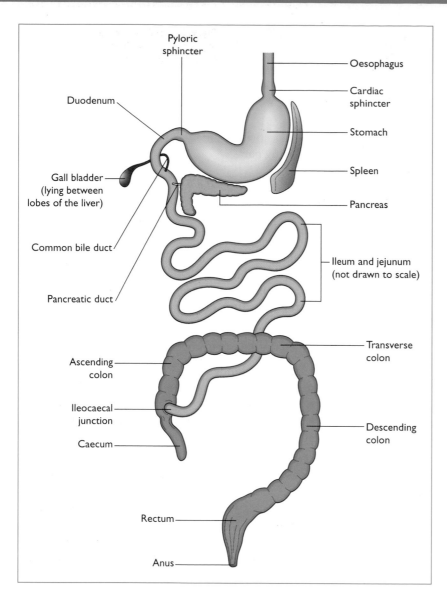

Fig. 9.2 The digestive tract removed from the body.

Labels in figure:
- Pyloric sphincter
- Oesophagus
- Cardiac sphincter
- Duodenum
- Stomach
- Gall bladder (lying between lobes of the liver)
- Spleen
- Pancreas
- Common bile duct
- Ileum and jejunum (not drawn to scale)
- Pancreatic duct
- Transverse colon
- Ascending colon
- Ileocaecal junction
- Caecum
- Descending colon
- Rectum
- Anus

THE ORAL CAVITY

The oral cavity (Fig. 9.3) is also known as the mouth or buccal cavity and contains the tongue, teeth and the salivary glands. The function of the oral cavity is as follows:

1. To pick up the food – known as *prehension* and involves the use of the lips and tongue
2. To break up the food into small boluses to aid swallowing – known as *mastication* or chewing and involves the use of the tongue, cheeks and teeth
3. Lubrication of the food with mucus and saliva making it easier to swallow
4. In omnivores and herbivores, digestion of carbohydrates begins in the mouth with the secretion of salivary enzymes. This does not occur in carnivores, e.g. dog and cat, as food is held in the mouth for a very short time before it is swallowed.

The oral cavity is formed by the following bones of the skull:

- The *incisive* bone and the *maxilla* form the upper jaw
- The *palatine* bone forms the roof of the mouth – the *hard palate*
- The *mandible* forms the lower jaw; the paired mandibles join in the midline at the *mandibular symphysis.*

The mandibles articulate with the *temporal* bones of the skull forming the *temporo-mandibular joint.* In carnivores the action of the joint is scissor-like to shear flesh off the bones of their prey.

The upper and lower jaws are linked by skin, forming the cheeks, under which lie the *muscles of mastication* (see Ch. 4). These muscles lie over the temporo-mandibular joint and give strength to the biting action. The entrance to the mouth is closed by the *lips,*

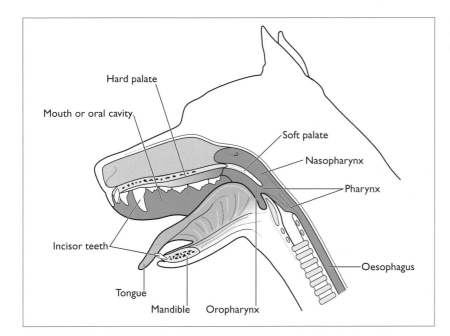

Fig. 9.3 Lateral view of the dog's head to show the oral cavity/digestive system.

composed of muscle covered in skin. The upper lip is split vertically by a division known as the *philtrum* (Fig. 8.1).

The entire oral cavity is lined by a layer of mucous membrane. It is reflected on to the jawbones, forming the *gums*. The mucous membrane covers the hard palate and extends over a flap of soft tissue at the back of the oral cavity – this is the *soft palate* which extends caudally between the oral and nasal cavities and divides the pharynx into the *oropharynx* and *nasopharynx* (Fig. 9.3).

The tongue

The functions of the tongue are:

1. To aid the ingestion of food
2. To carry the receptors (taste buds) for the sensation of taste or *gustation*
3. To help in the formation of a food bolus ready for swallowing
4. To groom the fur, particularly in cats
5. In thermoregulation – the tongue is used to apply saliva to the fur which smoothes it down into a thinner and cooler layer; in dogs, panting helps to cool the body
6. Vocalisation – production of sound involves complicated movements of the tongue and lips.

The tongue lies on the floor of the oral cavity and is made of *striated muscle fibres* running in all directions. This enables the tongue to make delicate movements. The muscles are attached at the *root* of the tongue to the hyoid bone (see Ch. 8) and to the sides of the mandibles. The tip of the tongue is unattached and very mobile.

The tongue is covered in mucous membrane. The dorsal surface is thicker and arranged in rough *papillae,*

APPLIED ANATOMY

In an anaesthetised animal, the sublingual vein may be used for intravenous injections or for collecting blood samples, while the sublingual artery may be used for monitoring the pulse rate.

which assist in control of the food bolus and in grooming. Some papillae are adapted to form taste buds, mainly found at the back of the tongue. Taste buds are well supplied with nerve fibres which carry information about taste to the forebrain (see Ch. 5). Running along the underside of the tongue are the paired *sublingual veins* and *arteries.*

The teeth

The teeth are hard structures embedded in the upper and lower jaw. Each jaw forms a *dental arch* – there are four dental arches in total. The teeth pierce the gums to sit in sockets or *alveoli.* The membrane covering the gums is known as the *gingival membrane* or *periodontal membrane.*

Structure

All teeth have a basic structure (Fig. 9.4). In the centre of each tooth is a *pulp cavity.* This contains blood capillaries and nerves which supply the growing tooth. In young animals the cavity is relatively large, but once the tooth is fully developed, it shrivels and contains only a small blood and nerve supply. After a tooth has stopped growing the only changes occurring will be due to wear.

Function

The teeth of a carnivore are adapted to shearing and tearing the flesh off the bones of their prey. There are food (particularly in dogs), fear, pain and irritant gases or other chemicals such as organophosphoruses. Salivation also often occurs just prior to vomiting and may be a warning sign to the owner!

The function of saliva is:

1. To lubricate the food, so making mastication and swallowing easier
2. Thermoregulation – evaporation of saliva from the tongue during panting or from the fur when applied during grooming causes cooling of blood in the underlying blood capillaries; this reduces the core temperature of the body
3. In omnivores and herbivores, secretions from the parotid gland contain amylase which begins carbohydrate digestion.

Pharynx

The pharynx forms a cross-over point between the respiratory and digestive systems. It is a muscular tube lined with mucous membrane, connecting the back of the nasal and oral cavities with the oesophagus and the larynx and trachea. The soft palate extends caudally towards the epiglottis of the larynx and divides the pharynx into the nasopharynx and oropharynx (Fig. 9.3). The walls of the pharynx contain diffuse areas of lymphoid tissue known as the *tonsils*. Their function is to protect the animal against disease (see Ch. 7). The most obvious are the palatine tonsils lying one on each side of the pharynx in a shallow recess. The *Eustachian* or *auditory tube* connects the pharynx to the middle ear. It enables the air pressure on either side of the tympanic membrane to equalise and thus maintains the flexibility and function of the ear drum (see Ch. 5).

The pharynx conveys food from the mouth into the oesophagus by means of a process known as *deglutition* or swallowing (Fig. 9.7). This occurs in the following stages:

1. The food is rolled into a bolus by the tongue and cheeks, and is passed to the back of the mouth by the base of the tongue.
2. The pharyngeal muscles contract and force the bolus towards the oesophagus.
3. At the same time, the epiglottis closes to prevent food entering the larynx.

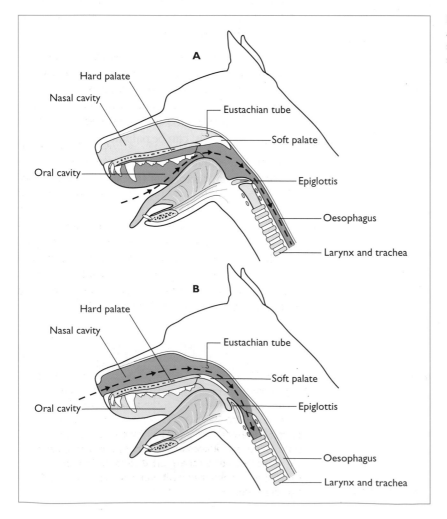

Fig. 9.7 Function of the pharynx. **A** Positions of structures during swallowing of food. **B** Position of structures during nose breathing.

A

Hard palate
Nasal cavity
Eustachian tube
Soft palate
Oral cavity
Epiglottis
Oesophagus
Larynx and trachea

B

Hard palate
Nasal cavity
Eustachian tube
Soft palate
Oral cavity
Epiglottis
Oesophagus
Larynx and trachea

4. A wave of muscular contraction – *peristalsis* – pushes the food down the oesophagus.
5. When the food has passed through the pharynx, the epiglottis falls open and respiration starts again.

Oesophagus

This is a simple tube which carries food from the pharynx to the stomach (Figs 9.1 and 9.2). In the neck, the oesophagus lies dorsal to the trachea and slightly to the left of it. It passes through the thoracic cavity, running within the mediastinum, dorsal to the heart base and between the two lungs. The oesophagus enters the abdominal cavity via the oesophageal hiatus of the diaphragm, which separates the thorax and abdomen.

The walls of the oesophagus are lined with *stratified squamous epithelium* arranged in longitudinal folds. This protects against damage by food and allows for widthways expansion as the boluses pass down. Within the walls are circular and longitudinal bands of smooth muscle fibres. Contraction of these muscles brings about a series of *peristaltic waves* which force the food along the tube (Fig. 9.8). Food can pass in the reverse direction – *antiperistalsis* – seen during vomiting. The average time taken for food to pass down the oesophagus is 15–30 seconds, but this depends on the type of food: liquids take a shorter time than dry foods.

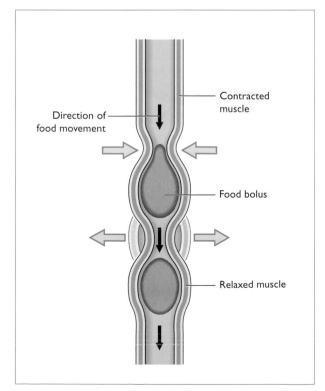

Fig. 9.8 Representation of peristalsis. Muscular contraction within the tube forces the food bolus along.

THE ABDOMINAL PART OF THE DIGESTIVE SYSTEM

The majority of the digestive tract lies within the abdominal cavity and can be divided into three parts:

1. *Stomach* – used to store and mix ingested food
2. *Small intestine* – the main site for enzymic digestion and the absorption of nutrients
3. *Large intestine* – the site for absorption of water, electrolytes and water soluble vitamins; any indigestible remains pass out of the anus as faeces.

Stomach

The stomach of the dog and cat is described as being *simple* and digestion is said to be *monogastric*. The functions of the stomach are:

1. To act as a reservoir for food – wild carnivores (particularly dogs) may only eat every 3–4 days and then rest while food slowly digests
2. To break up the food and mix it with gastric juices
3. To begin the process of protein digestion.

The stomach is a C-shaped sac-like organ lying on the left side of the cranial abdomen. Food enters from the oesophagus via the *cardiac sphincter* and leaves from the *pyloric sphincter* (Fig. 9.2). The inner curve of the sac is called the *lesser curvature* and the outer curve, the *greater curvature*. The entire organ is covered in a layer of visceral peritoneum or *mesentery,* as are all the organs in the abdominal cavity. The mesentery attached to the inner curvature is called the *lesser omentum,* while that attached to the greater curvature is called the *greater omentum*. The *spleen* lies within the

- *Pepsin* – converts protein molecules to peptides (smaller molecules) by a process known as hydrolysis.

The liquid food resulting from this process of gastric juice digestion is known as *chyme*.

Pancreatic juice

This secretion is produced by the exocrine part of the pancreas and occurs in response to the hormones *cholecystokinin* (produced by duodenal cells), *gastrin* (from the stomach wall) and to stimuli from the autonomic nervous system (see Ch. 6). It contains:

- *Bicarbonate* – neutralises the affects of the acid in the chyme, allowing other enzymes to work.
- *Digestive enzymes* – many are inactive precursors, which prevent autodigestion and destruction of the pancreas.
- *Proteases* – act on proteins and include:
  - *Trypsinogen,* converted to active trypsin by another enzyme, *enterokinase,* present in succus entericus
  - *Trypsin,* which activates other enzyme precursors. It acts on peptides and other proteins to produce amino acids. A trypsin inhibitor within the pancreas prevents spontaneous conversion of trypsinogen to trypsin and autodigestion.
- *Lipases* – activated by bile salts. They convert fats to fatty acids and glycerol.
- *Amylases* – act on starches, a form of plant carbohydrate, and convert them to maltose.

Bile salts

The presence of chyme in the duodenum causes the gall bladder to contract and produce bile. It emulsifies fat globules so that they have a larger surface area on which enzymes can act, and also activates lipases.

Intestinal juice

Secretion of intestinal juice is stimulated by the hormone *secretin* produced in response to the passage of chyme through the pyloric sphincter (see Ch. 6). The intestinal juices are produced by:

- Brunner's glands in the duodenum – the secretions are known as *succus entericus*
- Crypts of Leiberkuhn in the jejunum and ileum.

A number of enzymes are present, many of which are also produced by the pancreas:

- *Maltase* converts maltose to glucose
- *Sucrase* converts sucrose to glucose and fructose
- *Lactase* converts lactose to glucose and galactose
- *Enterokinase* converts trypsinogen to trypsin
- *Aminopeptidase* converts peptides to amino acids
- *Lipase* converts fats to fatty acids and glycerol.

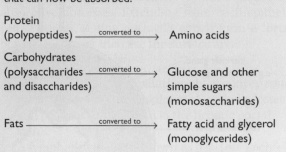

The result of the digestive process is that the basic constituents of food are converted into small molecules that can now be absorbed.

Protein (polypeptides) —— converted to ——▸ Amino acids

Carbohydrates (polysaccharides —— converted to ——▸ Glucose and other simple sugars (monosaccharides)
and disaccharides)

Fats —————— converted to ——▸ Fatty acid and glycerol (monoglycerides)

Absorption

The main site for absorption is the villi of the small intestine. The efficiency of the absorptive process is increased by:

- The long length of the small intestine
- The internal surface area (increased by the presence of the villi)
- Each villus is well supplied with blood capillaries and lacteals.

During absorption amino acids and simple sugars are absorbed by the blood capillaries and are carried by the hepatic portal vein to the liver. Fatty acids and glycerol are absorbed by the lacteals. They form a fatty milky liquid known as *chyle*, which is carried to the cisterna chyli, lying in the dorsal abdomen (see Ch. 7, Fig. 7.7). Here it is mixed with lymph and carried to the heart by the thoracic duct, where it joins the blood circulation.

Large intestine

This a short tube of a wider diameter than the small intestine. Each part has a similar structure to that of the small intestine. However, in the lumen, there are no villi and no digestive glands, but there are more goblet cells. These secrete mucus which lubricates the faeces as it passes through. The large intestine is divided into:

- *Caecum* – a short, blind-ending tube joining the ileum at its junction with the ascending colon: this is the *ileocaecal junction* (Fig. 9.2). In the carnivore it has no significant function.
- *Colon* – divided into the *ascending, transverse* and *descending colon* (Fig. 9.1) according to the relative position in the peritoneal cavity, but all are a continuation of the same organ. The descending colon is held close to the dorsal body wall by the *mesocolon.* Within the colon water, vitamins and electrolytes are absorbed ensuring that the body does not lose excessive water and become dehydrated.

■ *Rectum* – the part of the colon running through the pelvic cavity. It is held close to the dorsal body wall by connective tissue and muscle (Fig. 9.9).
■ *Anal sphincter* – this marks the end of the digestive tract. It is a muscular ring which controls the passage of faeces out of the body. It has two parts:
  – *Internal anal sphincter:* inner ring of smooth muscle; control is involuntary
  – *External anal sphincter:* outer ring of striated muscle; control is voluntary.

The lumen of the sphincter is constricted and lined with deep longitudinal folds of mucous membrane which stretch to allow the passage of bulky faeces.

Defaecation

The faecal mass passes through the large intestine by means of peristalsis, antiperistalsis, rhythmic segmentation and infrequent but strong contractions known as mass movements. These movements are involuntary, but as the faecal mass enters the pelvic cavity, stretching of the rectal wall stimulates voluntary straining. The anal sphincter, which is normally held tightly closed, relaxes, the abdominal muscles contract and the mass is forced out.

Composition of faeces

Normal faeces have a colour and smell that is characteristic of the species. They are described as being 'formed' – the water content is such that the faeces keep their shape (watery faeces do not). Normal faeces contain:

■ Water and fibre
■ Dead and living bacteria – normal commensals of the large intestine which may contribute to the smell
■ Sloughed intestinal cells
■ Mucus
■ Contents of anal sacs
■ Stercobilin – a pigment derived from bile that gives faeces their colour.

APPLIED ANATOMY

Lying between the two anal rings, in the '20 to 4' position, are the *anal sacs*. These are modified sebaceous glands which vary from pea to marble size depending on the species and breed of animal. Their secretions coat the faeces as it passes out and the characteristic smell is used by the animal for territorial scent marking, particularly in wild species. Impacted anal sacs may be a problem in dogs fed on softer diets.

APPLIED ANATOMY

The sequence of muscle contraction and nervous control involved in defaecation requires coordination by the nervous system. Any damage to the spinal cord, e.g. disc prolapse or severe trauma, may result in faecal incontinence or faecal retention.

Diarrhoea is 'frequent evacuation of watery faeces'. This is a common presenting sign. It may be acute or chronic and is an indication of some form of intestinal disturbance, e.g. maldigestion, malabsorption, increased peristalsis or gastrointestinal irritation. However, the most common cause of diarrhoea, in dogs especially, is dietary mismanagement. This can be easily corrected by starvation for 24 hours followed by a light diet of fish or chicken and rice for a further 24 hours.

The liver

The liver is the largest gland in the body and lies in the cranial abdomen. The cranial aspect is convex and is in contact with the diaphragm. The caudal aspect is concave and is in contact with the stomach, duodenum, and right kidney (Fig. 9.1). The liver is deep red in colour as it has a large volume of blood flowing through it. It is divided into several large *lobes,* in the centre of which is the *falciform ligament.* This is the remains of foetal blood vessels from the umbilicus and is of little significance in the adult animal (see Ch. 7). The *gall bladder* lies between the lobes in the centre of the caudal aspect. It stores bile, which pours into the duodenum via the common bile duct.

Histologically, the liver consists of thousands of cells known as *hepatocytes* (Fig. 9.13). These are responsible for all the many functions of the liver. The hepatocytes are arranged in hexagonal liver *lobules* surrounded by connective tissue. Running through the lobules between the hepatocytes are minute blood *sinusoids* carrying blood from the *hepatic portal vein.* Each hepatocyte is bathed in plasma, which percolates across the lobule to drain into the *central vein.* The central veins flow into the *hepatic vein* and so to the caudal vena cava. Thus the products of digestion are carried from the small intestine by the blood to every hepatocyte where they are used for metabolism. The liver tissue receives arterial blood in the *hepatic artery.*

Between the hepatocytes are tiny channels known as *bile canaliculi,* into which bile is secreted. The canaliculi form an interconnecting network that eventually drains into the gall bladder. There is no direct connection between the sinusoids and the canaliculi.

The liver has many functions and is essential to normal health.

1. *Carbohydrate metabolism* – glucose is a source of energy for the body but it can only be used by the cells in the presence of the hormone insulin, secreted by the pancreas. Excess glucose is stored as glycogen (glycogenesis) in the liver. This is broken down to release glucose (glycogenolysis) when blood glucose levels are low. In this way, the liver keeps blood glucose levels within a narrow range.

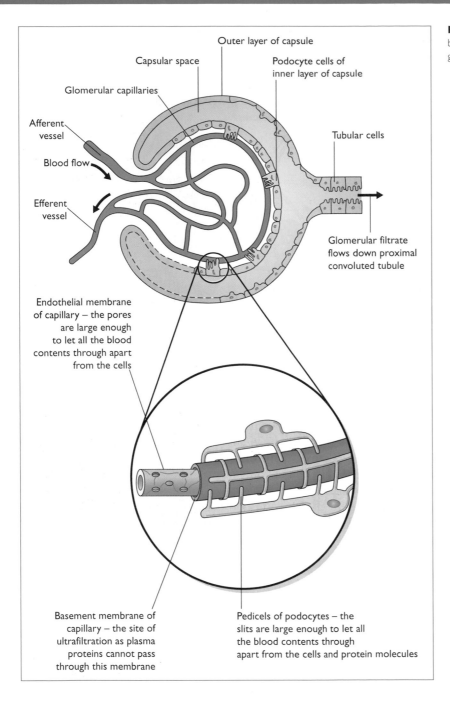

Outer layer of capsule

Capsular space

Podocyte cells of inner layer of capsule

Capsular space

Glomerular capillaries

Afferent vessel

Blood flow

Tubular cells

Efferent vessel

Glomerular filtrate flows down proximal convoluted tubule

Endothelial membrane of capillary – the pores are large enough to let all the blood contents through apart from the cells

Basement membrane of capillary – the site of ultrafiltration as plasma proteins cannot pass through this membrane

Pedicels of podocytes – the slits are large enough to let all the blood contents through apart from the cells and protein molecules

Blood enters the kidney and is carried to the capillaries forming the glomeruli.

Glomerulus

Blood pressure within each glomerulus is high because:

- The blood has come straight from the renal artery and the dorsal aorta, both of which carry blood under high pressure
- The smooth muscle in the walls of the arteriole leaving the glomerulus is able to constrict, under the control of the hormone *renin*, and thus regulate the pressure of blood in the glomerulus.

High pressure in the glomerulus forces fluid and small molecules out of the blood through the pores of the basement membrane into the capsule lumen. Larger sized particles such as red blood cells, plasma proteins and any substance bound to protein molecules, e.g. hormones are retained in the blood. This process is known as *ultrafiltration* and the filtrate is referred to as the *glomerular filtrate* or *primitive urine*. The glomerular filtrate is very dilute and contains 99% water and 1% chemical solutes.

Proximal convoluted tubule

Approximately 65% of all the resorptive processes take place here (Fig. 10.7). These are:

- *Reabsorption of water and sodium* – sodium (Na^+) and chloride (Cl^-) ions are actively reabsorbed from

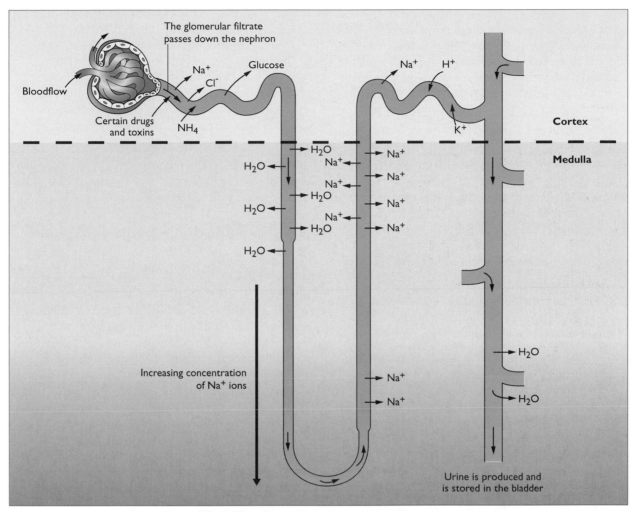

Fig. 10.7 Diagrammatic representation of the processes occurring in the different parts of the nephron.

APPLIED ANATOMY

In cases of diabetes mellitus, there is too much glucose in the blood (*hyperglycaemia*). This overflows into the glomerular filtrate and the tubules reabsorb it up to the limit of the renal threshold. The excess passes on down the tubules and out in the urine – *glucosuria* is a diagnostic sign of diabetes mellitus.

the filtrate into the blood. Water is reabsorbed by osmosis in response to the movement of Na$^+$ ions. 80% of all the Na$^+$ and Cl$^-$ ions in the filtrate are reabsorbed at this point.

■ *Reabsorption of glucose* – in the normal animal the glomerular filtrate contains glucose which is *all* reabsorbed back into the blood, so normal urine does not contain glucose. This reabsorption occurs up to a certain level referred to as the *renal threshold.*

■ *Concentration of nitrogenous waste* – the main waste product is urea, produced as a result of protein metabolism by the liver. Some diffuses back into

the blood from the tubule. Water reabsorption concentrates the levels of urea in the tubules.

■ *Secretion of toxins and certain drugs* – these are actively secreted into the filtrate. Penicillin, given therapeutically, is secreted from the blood and carried to the bladder in the urine. It is therefore a useful antibiotic for the treatment of bladder infections.

Loop of Henle

The function of the loop of Henle is to regulate the concentration and volume of the urine according to the status of the ECF. The glomerular filtrate flows first into the descending loop and then into the ascending loop, both of which lie in the medulla (Fig. 10.7).

■ *Descending loop of Henle* – the walls of the tubule are *permeable* to water but do not contain the mechanism to reabsorb Na$^+$. Water is drawn out of the tubule by osmosis – pulled by the concentration of Na$^+$ ions in the surrounding medullary tissue. The filtrate becomes more concentrated as it passes down the loop and reaches maximum concentration at the tip.

■ *Ascending loop of Henle* – the walls are *impermeable* to water but contain sodium pumps which actively reabsorb Na⁺ into the medullary tissue and capillaries. This draws water from the descending loop. Water cannot be drawn from the ascending loop as it is impermeable. The filtrate becomes less concentrated because the Na⁺ ions have been removed.

The net result of this mechanism is that the filtrate is the same concentration when it enters the loop of Henle as it is when it leaves and passes into the distal convoluted tubule, but it is reduced in volume as water has been removed. This water is reabsorbed into the blood – it has been conserved for use by the body. If the animal is dehydrated, more water is reabsorbed; if it is overhydrated, more water will be lost in the filtrate.

Distal convoluted tubule

It is here that the final adjustments are made to the chemical constituents of the urine in response to the status of the ECF. This is achieved by:

■ *Reabsorption of sodium (Na⁺) and secretion of potassium (K⁺)* – the amount of reabsorption of Na⁺ is much smaller than occurs in the proximal convoluted tubules. Reabsorption of water varies and is controlled by the hormone *aldosterone*, produced by the adrenal glands. K⁺ is excreted into the urine to replace the Na⁺ ions (Fig. 10.7).

■ *Regulation of acid/base balance by the excretion of hydrogen (H⁺) ions* – the normal pH of blood is 7.4.
  – If pH falls, i.e. the blood becomes more acid due to excess H⁺ ions, the kidney excretes H⁺ ions into the urine via the distal convoluted tubule. The pH of the blood returns to normal.
  – If pH rises, i.e. the blood becomes more alkaline due to reduced amounts of H⁺ ions, the kidney stops excreting H⁺ ions, retaining them in the blood. The pH of the blood falls to normal.

Collecting duct

Here the final adjustments are made to the volume of water in the urine in response to the status of the ECF (Fig. 10.7). The hormone *antidiuretic hormone* (ADH), produced by the posterior pituitary gland, is able to change the permeability of the duct walls to water.

APPLIED ANATOMY

Diuretics are drugs used to increase the volume of urine produced and so reduce the volume of fluid in the body. One of the most commonly used – frusemide – works by decreasing the reabsorption of Na⁺ from the distal convoluted tubules. This in turn decreases the reabsorption of water so the volume of urine increases.

■ If the animal is dehydrated, the volume of the plasma and ECF will be reduced. ADH will be produced, and the permeability of the collecting ducts to water will be increased. Water will be drawn through the walls by the high concentration of Na⁺ ions in the surrounding medullary tissue (secreted by the ascending loop of Henle), and into the plasma and ECF (Fig. 10.7).

As a result of the above processes, the ultrafiltrate that passed through the glomerular capsule has now become concentrated urine by the repeated effects of reabsorption and secretion.

Osmoregulation – control of renal function

Osmoregulation ensures that the volume of the plasma and the concentration of dissolved chemicals in the plasma and other tissue fluids remains constant. Homeostasis is maintained and the body can function normally. Several factors are involved in the control of osmoregulation (Table 10.1) and it is achieved in two ways:

1. Control of the amount of water lost from the body
2. Control of the amount of salt (NaCl) lost from the body.

Control of water loss

Water is lost by the healthy animal in urine, faeces, sweat and in respiration. Very small amounts may also be lost in vaginal secretions and tears. If this water loss is not replaced by food and drink, or if the water loss is excessive, e.g. in vomiting, diarrhoea or haemorrhage, the total volume of ECF falls and the animal is described as being *dehydrated.*

A dehydrated patient will show:

■ *Lowered blood pressure* – a fall in the volume of ECF results in a fall in blood plasma volume and consequently a fall in blood pressure
■ *A rise in osmotic pressure* – a fall in plasma volume results in a rise in the concentration of Na⁺ ions in the blood and as a result a rise in the osmotic pressure of the blood.

Note: *Osmotic pressure* is the pressure needed to prevent osmosis from occurring. It is dependent on the number of particles of undissolved molecules and ions in a solution. *Blood pressure* is the pressure exerted on the inside of the walls of the arterial blood vessels by the blood. It is detected by baroreceptors in the walls of the vessels.

In dehydration, osmoregulatory mechanisms will start to work (Fig. 10.8). The fall in blood pressure and rise in osmotic pressure ultimately result in an

Table 10.1 Factors involved in osmoregulation.

Controlling factor	Function
Renin (hormone)	Produced by the glomeruli of the kidney in response to low arterial pressure
Angiotensinogen (plasma protein)	Converted to angiotensin by the action of renin
Angiotensin (protein)	Causes vasoconstriction; stimulates the release of aldosterone from the adrenal cortex
Aldosterone (hormone – mineralocorticoid)	Secreted by the cortex of the adrenal gland; acts mainly on the distal convoluted tubules but has a lesser effect on the collecting ducts; regulates the reabsorption of Na+ ions
Antidiuretic hormone (ADH or vasopressin)	Secreted by the posterior pituitary gland; mainly affects the collecting ducts by changing their permeability to water; also has an effect on the distal convoluted tubules
Baroreceptors	Found in the walls of the blood vessels; monitor arterial blood pressure
Osmoreceptors	Found in the hypothalamus; monitor the osmotic pressure of the plasma; affect the thirst centre of the brain and influence the secretion of ADH

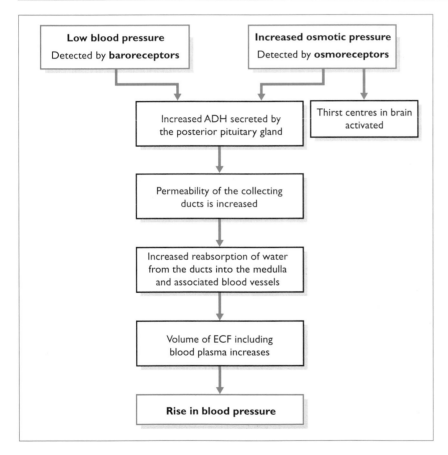

Fig. 10.8 Mechanism controlling the amount of water lost from the kidney.

increase in the reabsorption of water from the collecting ducts, under the control of the hormone ADH (see Ch. 6). The osmoreceptors also stimulate the thirst centre in the brain and the animal feels the need to drink. Both of these pathways result in a rise in plasma volume and an increase in arterial blood pressure. Dehydrated animals should be given fluid parenterally (intravenously) or, in less severe cases, provided with access to drinking water. They will excrete *reduced* quantities of *concentrated* urine.

Raised blood pressure will result in the opposite effect, and the animal will produce *increased* quantities of more *dilute* urine.

Control of sodium levels
Sodium is taken into the body in the form of salt (NaCl) in food. It is lost in sweat, faeces and urine. Sodium is found in the ionised form Na+ in all the body fluid compartments and plays a fundamental part in determining arterial blood pressure. High Na+ levels in

as the *preprostatic urethra* which is not found in the dog. The urethra continues caudally and opens to the outside in the perineal area, ventral to the anus. There is no penile urethra lying outside the pelvic cavity. Close to the end of the urethra are the openings from the paired *bulbourethral* glands.

From the point at which the deferent ducts join it, the urethra conveys both urine and sperm to the outside of the body.

URINATION AND URINALYSIS

Micturition

Micturition is the act of expelling urine from the bladder. It is normally a reflex activity but can be over-ridden by voluntary control from the brain. The steps involved are:

■ Bladder distends with urine formed by the kidneys
■ Stretch receptors in the smooth muscle of the bladder wall are stimulated and send nerve impulses to centres in the spinal cord

■ Nerve impulses are transmitted via parasympathetic nerves back to the smooth muscle, and initiate contraction
■ Nerve impulses also stimulate relaxation in the internal bladder sphincter and urine is expelled.

If it is inappropriate for the animal to micturate, the brain over-rides the reflex pathway and prevents the bladder sphincter from relaxing. At a more appropriate time, the brain stimulates both the external and internal sphincters: they relax and urine is released. Voluntary control develops as the young animal matures – in puppies and kittens it is not fully developed until the animal is about 10 weeks old.

Urinalysis

As urine is derived from the ultrafiltrate of plasma, it reflects the health status of the whole animal and is a useful diagnostic tool. Normal urine contains only water, salts and urea. The clinical parameters used to evaluate a sample of urine are shown in the Table 10.2.

🔑 KEY POINTS

■ The functional unit of the kidney is the nephron; each kidney contains many thousands of nephrons.

■ Each nephron is made of several parts, each of which has a role in modifying the glomerular filtrate.

■ Within the glomerular capsule of the nephrons, blood passes over a fine filter. Water and very small particles are removed – this is known as ultrafiltration and forms what is known as the glomerular filtrate.

■ Large particles such as red blood cells and plasma proteins remain in the blood.

■ The very dilute glomerular filtrate passes down the nephrons and undergoes a series of modifications which result in the formation of urine. The final volume of the urine is significantly reduced and reflects the status of the extracellular fluid of the body.

■ The function of the kidney is to regulate the volume and the osmotic concentration of the body fluids so that they remain constant – this is one of the homeostatic mechanisms of the body and is essential if the body is to function normally.

■ The kidney is also responsible for the excretion of nitrogenous waste in the urine.

■ Urine is stored in the bladder and removed from the body via the urethra.

■ Urine samples can provide useful diagnostic information.

Table 10.2 Normal values shown by the urine of the dog and cat.

Clinical parameter	Normal value	Comments
Daily volume	Dog: 20–100 mL/kg body weight	*Polyuria* – increased volume of urine
		Oliguria – reduced volume of urine
	Cat: 10–12 mL/kg body weight	*Anuria* – absence of urine
Appearance	Clear, yellow, characteristic smell	Tomcat urine has an unpleasant strong smell; old samples smell ammoniacal
pH	5–7	Carnivorous diet produces acid urine; herbivorous diet produces alkaline urine
Specific gravity (s.g.)	Dog: 1.016–1.060	Reflects the concentration of urine; exercise, high environmental temperatures and dehydration will cause a rise in s.g.
	Cat: 1.020–1.040	
Protein	None	*Proteinuria* – presence of protein.
		May indicate damage to nephrons, chronic renal failure, inflammation of the urinary tract
Blood	None	*Haematuria* – presence of blood
		Haemoglobinuria – presence of haemoglobin, due to rupture of red cells
		May indicate damage or infection to the urinary tract.
Glucose	None	*Glucosuria* – presence of glucose
		May indicate diabetes mellitus; levels of glucose in the filtrate exceed the renal threshold and excess is excreted in the urine
Ketones	None	*Ketonuria* – presence of ketones
		May be accompanied by acid pH and smell of 'peardrops' in urine and on the breath
Bile	None	*Bilirubinuria* – presence of bile
		Indicator of some form of liver disease
Crystals and casts	In small quantities, these may be considered to be normal	Crystalline or colloidal material coalesce to form a cast of the renal tubules and are flushed out by the urine; in large quantities crystals may form calculi or uroliths and block the tract

11 THE REPRODUCTIVE SYSTEM

Reproduction is the means by which a species is able to perpetuate itself. If animals lived for ever, there would be no need for another generation to take over from previous ones; in reality, all animals become old or 'worn out' and die and must be replaced if the species is not to become extinct.

All species of mammals have evolved separate sexes and reproduce *sexually*. This is in contrast to less highly evolved species, which may reproduce *asexually* – producing offspring that are identical to the parent. Sexual reproduction involves the transfer of genetic material. Specialised germ cells – *spermatozoa* and *ova* – develop in the male or female animal and fuse to form a single-celled *zygote*. The zygote undergoes cell division to form the *embryo*. The

offspring resulting from sexual reproduction are genetically different from each other and from their parents.

The reproductive system shares part of its structure with the urinary system and the combined systems may be referred to as the *urogenital system*.

MALE REPRODUCTIVE SYSTEM

The male dog is known as a dog; the male cat is known as a tomcat. The reproductive system of the dog and the tomcat are generally similar – any differences will be described where appropriate (Figs 11.1 and 11.2). The parts of the male reproductive tract are:

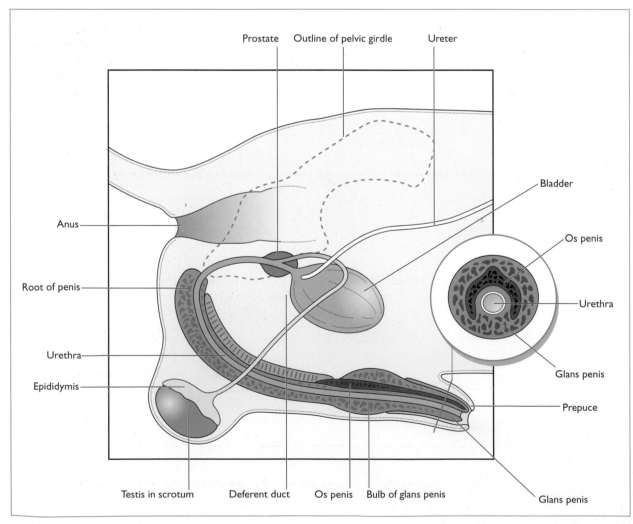

Fig. 11.1 Reproductive system of the dog.

- Testis
- Epididymis
- Deferent duct, also called the vas deferens
- Urethra
- Penis
- Prostate gland – an accessory gland
- Bulbourethral gland – an accessory gland seen only in the tomcat.

The testis

The testis is the male gonad, with functions as follows:

- To produce spermatozoa (sperm) by the process of spermatogenesis; these fertilise the ova produced by the female
- To produce fluid to transport the sperm from the testes into the female tract and to aid their survival
- To secrete the hormone testosterone which influences spermatogenesis, the development of male secondary sexual characteristics and male behaviour patterns (see Ch. 6).

There is a pair of testes which, in the adult animal, lie outside the body cavity in the *scrotum.* – a sac of relatively hairless and often pigmented skin. Spermatogenesis occurs most efficiently at temperatures below that of the core body temperature, so the testes are carried outside the body cavity in a cooler environment. In the dog, the scrotum lies between the hindlegs; in the cat it is attached to the perineum, ventral to the anus.

Internally, the sac is divided into two, each part containing one testis; the left testis often hangs lower than the right one. Within the wall of the scrotum is the *Dartos muscle.* In cold weather this contracts and thickens the scrotal skin, raising the temperature; in warm weather, the muscle relaxes and the scrotum becomes thinner and thus cooler. A constant temperature for spermatogenesis is therefore maintained.

Each testis is an oval-shaped structure wrapped in a double layer of peritoneum known as the *tunica vaginalis* (Fig. 11.3). The testis tissue consists of numerous blind-ending tubules known as *seminiferous tubules* which are lined by two types of cells:

1. *Spermatogenic cells* – these divide by *meiosis* to produce immature sperm or spermatids; each spermatid contains the haploid number of chromosomes (see Ch. 1)
2. *Sertoli cells* – these secrete *oestrogen* and nutrients which prolong the survival of the sperm.

Lying between the tubules are the *cells of Leydig* or *interstitial cells.* They secrete *testosterone* and are under the control of *interstitial cell stimulating hormone* (ICSH) (see Ch. 6), produced by the anterior pituitary gland.

The coiled seminiferous tubules make up most of the testicular tissue and eventually combine to form slightly larger *efferent ducts.* These drain into the *epididymis,* lying along the dorsolateral border of the testis. The *cauda epididymis* or *tail* is attached to the

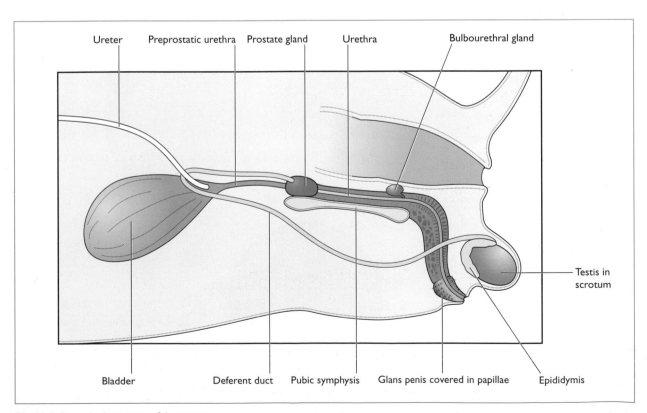

Fig. 11.2 Reproductive system of the tomcat.

caudal extremity of the testis and is the point at which the temperature of the testis is lowest. It is here that sperm are stored and undergo a period of maturation ready for fertilisation (Fig. 11.4).

The blood supply to the testis is via the *testicular artery*. This leaves the dorsal aorta in the abdomen, just caudal to the renal artery. As it enters the scrotum, the testicular artery runs alongside the epididymis and then divides to form the convoluted *pampiniform plexus.* This complicated capillary network ensures that the blood is cooled before it enters the testicular tissue.

Testicular descent

In the early embryo, the undifferentiated gonads develop inside the abdomen close to the kidney. In the male, the gonad becomes the testis and a band of tissue known as the *gubernaculum* forms and runs from the caudal end of each testis to the inside of the developing scrotal sac. During late gestation, the testes are pulled caudally by the contraction of the gubernaculum and they migrate through the abdomen. The testes leave the abdominal cavity via the *inguinal canal* – a channel between the fibres of the external abdominal

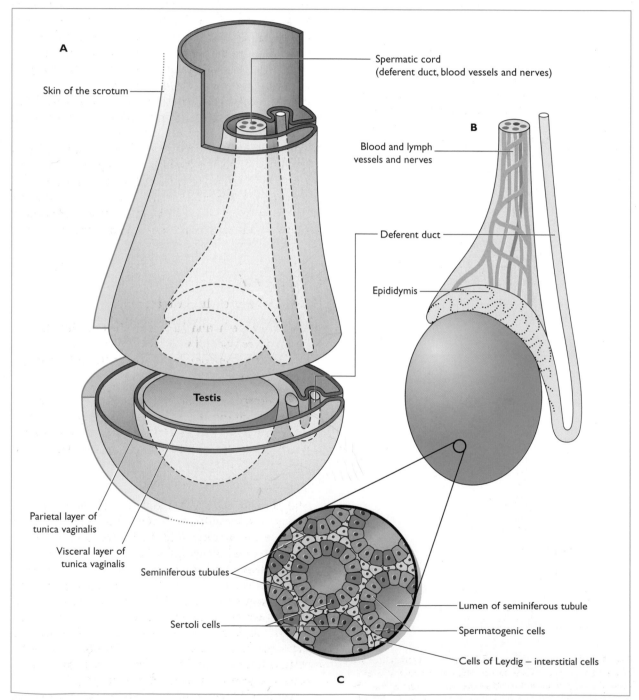

Fig. 11.3 A Testis within scrotum. **B** Scrotum removed. **C** Cross-section through the seminiferous tubules.

oblique muscle in the groin or inguinal area (see Ch. 4). As each testis with its associated blood capillaries, nerve and deferent duct passes through the inguinal canal into the scrotum, it becomes wrapped in a double fold of peritoneum which forms the tunica vaginalis (Fig. 11.3).

The testes begin their descent into the scrotum during early neonatal life and should be palpable within the scrotum by 12 weeks of age in the puppy and 10–12 weeks in the kitten. Failure of the testes to descend is described as *cryptorchidism;* the testes may be retained in the abdomen or within the inguinal canal.

APPLIED ANATOMY

Retention of the testis may be a hereditary condition and affected dogs should not be used for breeding. Bilaterally cryptorchid dogs are usually sterile but may have normal sexual libido (desire). As the dog grows older, the retained testis is more likely to develop a Sertoli cell tumour.

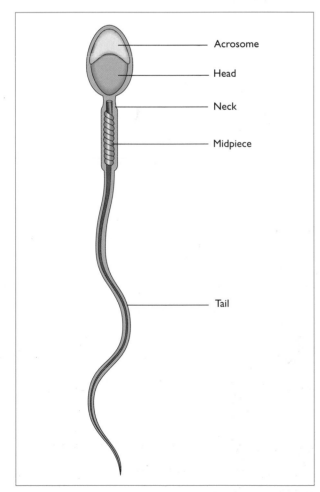

Fig. 11.4 A normal spermatozoon. The acrosome protects the head of the sperm and contains emzymes which aid penetration of the ovum. The head contains the haploid number of chromosomes. The midpiece contains enzymes and mitochondria to provide energy for movement. The tail produces a powerful propulsive force.

- *Monorchid* – term used when one testis is retained.
- *Bilateral cryptorchid* – term used when both testes are retained.

Deferent duct

The epididymis continues as the *deferent duct* (also called the *vas deferens* or *ductus deferens;* Figs 11.1 and 11.2) which passes out of the scrotum into the abdominal cavity via the inguinal canal within the *spermatic cord.* The spermatic cord is wrapped in the tunica vaginalis and also contains the testicular artery and vein and the testicular nerve. Lying within the cord is a strip of muscle derived from the internal abdominal oblique muscle and known as the *cremaster muscle.* Contraction of this muscle raises the testis closer to the body in response to cold and works in conjunction with the Dartos muscle to maintain a constant temperature for the testes.

During ejaculation, the sperm and fluid produced in the seminiferous tubules are propelled along the epididymis and up the deferent duct, which joins the urethra. At this junction, the walls of the deferent ducts are thickened and glandular; the whole area is surrounded by the *prostate gland* (Figs 11.1 and 11.2).

The penis

The functions of the penis are to:

- Convey sperm and fluids from the testis into the female reproductive tract during mating
- Convey urine from the bladder to the outside via the urethra.

The urethra runs through the centre of the penis and extends from the bladder to the tip of the penis. It is shared by both the reproductive and urinary systems (see Ch. 10). The penis of the dog and the cat are anatomically different.

The dog

The penis runs from the ischial arch of the pelvis, passes cranioventrally along the perineum and between the hindlegs (Fig. 11.5). The urethra lies in the centre and is surrounded by a layer of cavernous erectile tissue known as the *corpus spongiosum penis.* This is expanded proximally into the *bulb of the penis* and, towards the tip, as the *glans penis.* Surrounding this and serving to attach the penis to the ischial arch is a pair of erectile tissue *crura* (sing. *crus*), known as the *corpus cavernosum penis.* These form the *root* of the penis at its attachment to the ischial arch. The urethra runs in a groove between the two crura.

Within the tissue of the glans penis is a tunnel-shaped bone, the *os penis,* whose function is to aid

APPLIED ANATOMY

Cavernous erectile tissue is made of connective tissue perforated by 'caverns' lined by endothelium. During sexual excitement these caverns fill with blood under pressure and the tissue becomes engorged and erect.

entry of the penis into the vagina of the bitch during the early stages of mating when erection is only partially complete. The canine os penis lies *dorsal* to the urethra, which runs through the 'tunnel' in the bone. At this point the urethra cannot expand and this can be a common site for urethral blockage with urinary calculi.

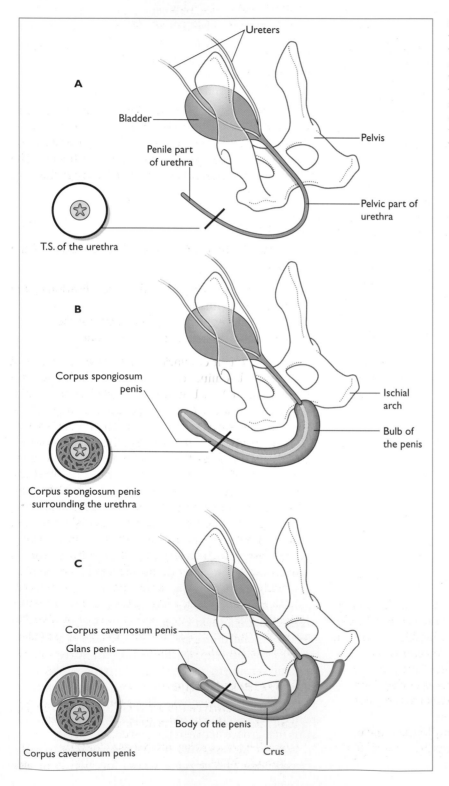

A

Ureters

Bladder

Penile part of urethra

Pelvis

Pelvic part of urethra

T.S. of the urethra

B

Corpus spongiosum penis

Ischial arch

Bulb of the penis

Corpus spongiosum penis surrounding the urethra

C

Corpus cavernosum penis

Glans penis

Body of the penis

Corpus cavernosum penis

Crus

Fig. 11.5 Structure of the penis in three layers, with transverse sections through the urethra. **A** Shows the urethra only. **B** Shows the urethra with the layer of cavernous erectile tissue surrounding it: the corpus spongiosum penis. **C** Shows the corpus cavernosum penis, which forms the two crura and attaches the penis to the ischial arch.

The distal part of the penis is contained within a sheath of hairy skin known as the *prepuce*. This is suspended from the ventral abdominal wall and covers and protects the penis. It is lined with mucous membrane and is well supplied with lubricating glands. During mating, the prepuce is pushed back to reveal the glans penis. Afterwards, the *retractor penis muscle* pulls the penis back into the prepuce.

The tomcat

The main parts of the penis are similar to those of the dog, except that the cat penis is shorter and points backwards – the external opening is ventral to the anus (Fig. 11.2). The glans penis is covered with tiny barbs, which elicit a pain reflex as the male withdraws from the female after mating. This stimulates the nerve pathway to the hypothalamus, resulting in ovulation approximately 36 hours later – known as *induced ovulation*. The *os penis* lies *ventral* to the urethra in the cat. During sexual excitement, the penis engorges and points cranioventrally so that the mating position in cats is similar to that seen in the dog.

Accessory glands

The function of the accessory glands is to secrete *seminal fluids* which:

- Increase the volume of the ejaculate to aid the passage of sperm into the female tract
- Provide the correct environment for sperm survival
- Neutralise the acidity of the urine within the urethra.

There are two types of glands (Figs 11.1 and 11.2):

1. *Prostate gland* – the gland is bilobed and lies on the floor of the pelvis, surrounding the urethra. In the dog, it is close to the neck of the bladder; in the cat, there is a short *preprostatic urethra* cranial to the gland (see Ch. 10). Enlargement of the prostate may obstruct the passage of faeces as they pass down the rectum, which lies dorsal to the gland within the pelvic cavity.
2. *Bulbourethral glands* – found only in the tomcat. They lie on either side of the urethra, cranial to the ischial arch (Fig. 11.2).

FEMALE REPRODUCTIVE SYSTEM

The female dog is known as a bitch; the female cat is known as a queen. The parts of the female reproductive system are:

- Ovary
- Uterine tube or oviduct
- Uterus – uterine horns and body
- Cervix
- Vagina
- Vestibule
- Vulva.

The reproductive tract of the bitch and queen are similar and vary only in size (Fig. 11.6). The tract is designed to carry several fetuses during a single pregnancy and is said to be *bicornuate* (two horns). The bitch and the queen bear litters of young: they are *multiparous*.

The ovary

The ovary is the female gonad. The functions of the ovary are:

- To produce ova or eggs ready for fertilisation by the sperm of the male
- To act as an endocrine gland, secreting the hormones oestrogen and progesterone.

There is a pair of ovaries, one lying on each side of the dorsal abdominal cavity, caudal to the kidney (see Ch. 10, Fig. 10.2). The ovary is held close to the kidney by the *ovarian (suspensory) ligament* (Fig. 11.7). The ovary is suspended from the dorsal body wall by part of the visceral peritoneum called the *mesovarium*, which also encloses the infundibulum of the uterine tube. Part of the mesovarium forms a pocket-like structure known as the *ovarian bursa* which completely covers the ovary. Within this is a small opening allowing ova to leave the ovary – this is a potential means of entry of infection into the peritoneal cavity.

The tissue of the ovary consists of a framework of connective tissue, smooth muscle and blood capillaries, within which are a large number of germ cells and developing follicles (Fig. 11.8). In an immature animal, each ovary is oval with a smooth outline, but as sexual maturity approaches, the ovary becomes nodular as the follicles enlarge.

The uterine tube

This is also known as the *oviduct* or *Fallopian tube* (Fig. 11.6). The functions of the uterine tubes are:

- To collect ova as they are released from the Graafian follicles

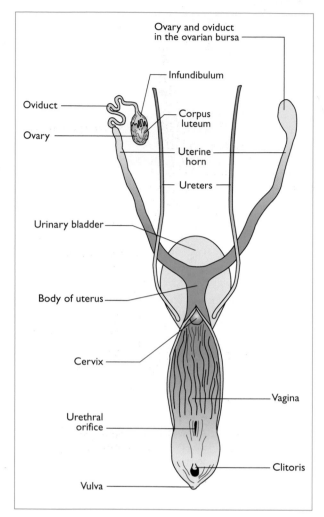

Fig. 11.6 Dorsal view of the reproductive system of the bitch. (Reprinted from Clinical Anatomy and Physiology for Veterinary Technicians, T Colville and JM Bassett, p 330, Copyright 2002, with permission from Elsevier Science.)

The uterus

The uterus is Y-shaped structure lying in the midline of the dorsal abdomen (Fig. 11.6). During pregnancy, the weight of the conceptuses pulls the uterus ventrally and at full term it occupies the greater part of the abdomen. The function of the uterus is:

- To provide a receptacle in which the embryos can develop into full-term fetuses
- To provide the correct environment for the survival of the embryos
- To provide the means whereby the developing embryos can receive nutrients from the dam – this is made possible by the *placenta.*

The uterus consists of two parts. A pair of *uterine horns* lead from the uterine tubes. Each horn is about five times the length of the uterine body and, during pregnancy, contains the developing embryos. The two horns join to form a short central *body.*

The wall of the uterus has three layers:

1. *Endometrium* – lining of columnar mucous membrane, glandular tissue and blood vessels. During pregnancy this thickens to provide nutrition for the embryo before implantation and to support the developing placenta.
2. *Myometrium* – layers of smooth muscle which produces strong contractions during parturition.
3. *Mesometrium* or *broad ligament* – this fold of the visceral peritoneum suspends the uterus from the dorsal body wall and is continuous with the mesovarium and mesosalpinx.

The cervix

The cervix is a short thick-walled muscular sphincter that connects the uterine body with the vagina (Fig. 11.6). Running through the centre is a narrow *cervical canal* which is normally tightly closed and relaxes only to allow the passage of sperm or fetuses. During pregnancy, the canal is blocked by a mucoid plug which protects the conceptuses from infection. In the non-pregnant animal, the cervix lies in the pelvic cavity, but

APPLIED ANATOMY

Ovariohysterectomy, more commonly called 'spaying', is performed by the veterinary surgeon to prevent unwanted pregnancies and oestrous cycles. The surgical procedure involves the complete removal of the reproductive tract from the ovaries to a point just cranial to the cervix. Ligation of the major blood vessels is essential, particularly if the procedure is performed during oestrus or pregnancy as the vessels may be extremely well developed.

- To convey the ova from the ovaries to the uterine horns
- To provide the correct environment for the survival of both the ova and sperm.

Each uterine tube is a narrow convoluted structure lying close to the ovary (Fig. 11.7). The open end is funnel-shaped and known as the *infundibulum.* It is fringed with finger-like processes known as *fimbriae,* which spread over the surface of the ovary to capture ova as they are released. The ova pass down the lumen of the tube, which is lined with ciliated columnar epithelium. The cilia propel the ova along the tube towards the uterine horns. The uterine tube is suspended by part of the visceral peritoneum known as the *mesosalpinx.*

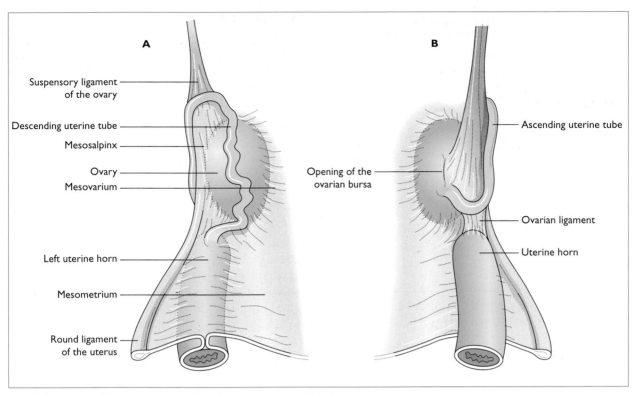

Fig. 11.7 Anatomy of the ovarian region of the bitch. **A** Lateral view. **B** Medial view.

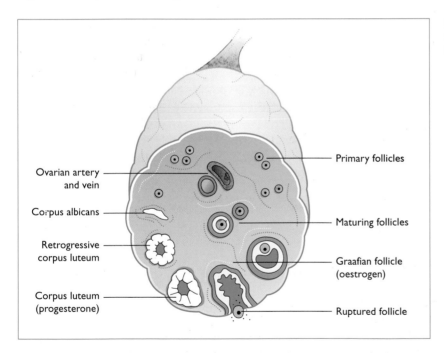

Fig. 11.8 Longitudinal section through an ovary to show ovarian activity.

during pregnancy the weight of the conceptuses pulls the cervix cranially and ventrally over the edge of the pelvic brim.

Blood supply to the reproductive tract

The blood vessels run within the mesovarium, mesosalpinx and mesometrium. They are:

- *Ovarian artery* – arises from the dorsal aorta just caudal to the renal artery and supplies the ovary, uterine tube and uterine horn
- *Uterine artery* – anastomoses with the ovarian artery and supplies the caudal part of the tract. It can be seen as a relatively large artery running on either side of the cervix.

The vagina and vestibule

The vagina and vestibule form a channel leading to the external opening of the reproductive tract – the *vulva*. The vagina leads from the cervix to the *external urethral orifice* – the point at which the urethra joins the reproductive tract. The vestibule leads from the external urethral orifice to the vulva and is shared by both the urinary and reproductive tracts.

The lumen is lined by *stratified squamous epithelium* which undergoes hormonal changes during the oestrous cycle. The lining epithelium is folded longitudinally to allow widthways expansion during parturition and is surrounded by layers of smooth muscle. These are very strong and during canine mating they tighten on the penis of the male and maintain the 'tie'.

The vulva

The vulva marks the external opening of the urogenital tract. It consists of two parts:

1. *The labiae* – two vertical lips joined dorsally and ventrally; the vertical slit between them is known as the *vulval cleft*. They are normally held closed to prevent the entry of infection. During proestrus and oestrus in the bitch, the labiae enlarge, but this is not seen in the oestrous cycle of the queen.
2. *The clitoris* – a knob-like structure of cavernous erectile tissue lying in the *clitoral fossa* just inside the ventral angle of the vulval cleft. It is the equivalent of the male penis.

The mammary glands

Although these are not strictly part of the reproductive tract, they are essential to reproduction in the mammal. The presence of mammary glands is the defining characteristic of the class Mammalia. All mammals feed their young on milk produced by the glands during a process known as *lactation*.

Mammary glands are modified cutaneous glands. In the dog and cat, they are present in both sexes but are rudimentary in the male. The glands lie externally on the ventral wall of the abdomen and thorax, on either side of the midline.

> ■ The bitch has five pairs of mammary glands.
> ■ The queen has four pairs of mammary glands.

Each gland consists of glandular tissue embedded in connective tissue and lined by a secretory epithelium (Fig. 11.9). The milk produced drains through a network of sinuses that eventually form *teat canals*. These open on to the surface of each teat, known as a *teat orifice*. Each gland has one teat but each teat has several orifices.

Lactation

This is the production of milk and normally occurs during pregnancy. It is influenced by three hormones:

1. *Progesterone* – secreted by the corpus luteum within the ovary and causes enlargement of the mammary glands during pregnancy
2. *Prolactin* – secreted by the anterior pituitary gland in the last third of pregnancy and stimulates the production of milk
3. *Oxytocin* – secreted by the posterior pituitary gland during the last hours of pregnancy and enables the glands to release or 'let down' the milk in response to suckling by the neonate.

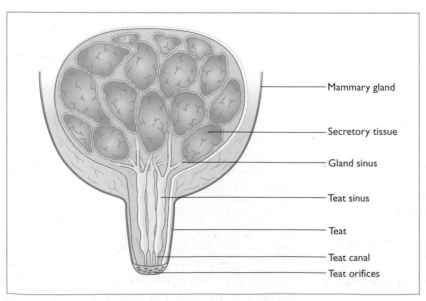

Mammary gland

Secretory tissue

Gland sinus

Teat sinus

Teat

Teat canal

Teat orifices

Fig. 11.9 Section through a mammary gland.

Composition of milk

This varies between different species and is an important consideration when feeding orphaned animals. The milk produced by the bitch and the queen is more concentrated and contains more protein and twice as much fat as cow's milk. The average composition of milk is shown in Table 11.1.

The first milk secreted by the dam following parturition is known as *colostrum*. It is rich in maternal antibodies, which provide the neonate with immunity to diseases to which the dam has been exposed. It is essential that the neonate takes in colostrum within the first 24 hours of life. During this time, the protein antibodies can be absorbed by the small intestine without being digested. After 24 hours, normal protein digestion starts and the antibodies are broken down and destroyed. After a few days, production of colostrum stops and the composition of the milk remains constant.

THE OESTROUS CYCLE

The oestrous cycle is the rhythmic cycle of events that occurs in sexually mature non-pregnant female mammals and includes limited periods of sexual receptivity known as *oestrus*. The function of the oestrous cycle is:

- To produce ova ready for fertilisation by the male spermatozoa
- To prepare the female reproductive tract to receive the fertilised ova
- To initiate behavioural patterns in the female that indicate to the male that she is receptive to mating
- To stimulate the female to stand still and allow the male to mate with her.

For the oestrous cycle to achieve the aim of a fertile mating, the timing of all interrelated components must coincide. The pattern and timing of the oestrous cycle varies between species – the cycle shown by the bitch is different to that shown by the queen.

Each cycle is divided into phases of varying lengths. These are:

1. Proestrus – period in which the reproductive tract is under the influence of oestrogen
2. Oestrus – period during which the female will allow herself to be mated
3. Metoestrus – also called dioestrus; period during which the tract is under the influence of progesterone
4. Anoestrus – period between cycles during which there is little or no ovarian activity.

During the oestrous cycle simultaneous changes occur in:

Table 11.1 Average composition of milk.

Constituent	Quantity
Water	70–90%
Fat	0–30%
Protein	1–15%
Carbohydrate	3–7%
Minerals	1.5–1%: calcium phosphate, magnesium, sodium, potassium and chloride
	Milk is deficient in iron and copper; traces of iodine, cobalt, tin and silica are present
Vitamins	A,B$_2$,B$_5$,E,K Milk is low in vitamins C and D

- The ovary and reproductive tract – includes ovulation
- The endocrine system – interaction between the hormones oestrogen, progesterone, follicle stimulating hormone and luteinising hormone
- The animal's behavioural patterns.

Ovary and reproductive tract

At birth, the ovary contains all the *germ cells* that the animal will ever need; these act as a reservoir from which the *primary follicles* develop. At the onset of puberty or sexual maturity, several primary follicles develop to form ripe *Graafian follicles*. In multiparous species, there will be many follicles, divided between the two ovaries, but not necessarily equally. Each Graafian follicle consists of an ovum formed by the process of meiosis and containing the haploid number of chromosomes (see Ch. 1). This is suspended in fluid and surrounded by an outer layer of follicular cells. The Graafian follicle secretes the hormone *oestrogen* (Fig. 11.8).

When the follicle has reached full size, it ruptures to release the ovum – the process of *ovulation*. The ovum passes down the uterine tube and the remaining follicular tissue becomes reorganised to form the *corpus luteum*. The corpus luteum secretes the hormone *progesterone*.

Within the reproductive tract, the uterine walls become thickened and more glandular to create a suitable environment for implantation of the fertilised ova. The vaginal epithelium also changes and the blood-stained discharge seen in proestrus in the bitch comes from the lining of the vagina. Study of the epithelial cells in vaginal smears at intervals during proestrus can be used to gauge the correct time for mating – this technique is known as *exfoliative cytology*.

Hormonal changes

Ovulation and the oestrous cycle are associated with a cycle of interrelated hormonal changes in the ovary and anterior pituitary gland (see Ch. 6, Fig. 6.4):

1. External stimuli such as increasing daylength or a rise in environmental temperature stimulate the hypothalamus in the forebrain. This releases *gonadotrophin releasing hormone (GRH)*, which acts on the anterior pituitary gland.
2. The anterior pituitary secretes *follicle stimulating hormone* (FSH), which stimulates a few primary follicles in the ovary to ripen into Graafian follicles.
3. The ripening follicles secrete increasing levels of *oestrogen*, which:
   – Produces the behaviour of the female seen during proestrus
   – Prepares the reproductive tract for mating
   – Stimulates the secretion of *luteinising hormone* (LH) from the anterior pituitary gland
   – Inhibits further secretion of FSH.
4. As a result of FSH inhibition, oestrogen levels begin to fall. LH acts on the ripe follicles and brings about ovulation. After the release of the ovum, the remaining follicular tissue becomes luteinised, i.e. converted into the corpus luteum.
5. The corpus luteum begins to secrete *progesterone*. The increasing levels of progesterone and the decreasing levels of oestrogen stimulate mating behaviour in the bitch – she will allow the male to mount her.
6. Progesterone is the dominant hormone during pregnancy. It:
   – Prepares the reproductive tract to receive the fertilised ova
   – Causes enlargement of the mammary glands
   – Inhibits the secretion of GRH from the hypothalamus, which inhibits FSH output and prevents the development of any more follicles.

If the animal has not conceived, the corpus luteum regresses and the cycle begins again.

APPLIED ANATOMY

Pseudopregnancy (false pregnancy or pseudocyesis) is linked to the fact that the corpus luteum of the bitch remains in the ovary for about 6–7 weeks, *whether she is pregnant or not.* Progesterone levels remain high and produce symptoms such as maternal behaviour, enlargement of mammary glands and lactation. Progesterone levels are normally high in all bitches, but clinical signs only occur in certain bitches.

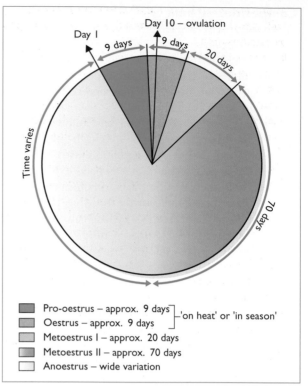

Pro-oestrus – approx. 9 days ⎤
Oestrus – approx. 9 days ⎦ –'on heat' or 'in season'
Metoestrus I – approx. 20 days
Metoestrus II – approx. 70 days
Anoestrus – wide variation

Fig. 11.10 Phases of the oestrus cycle of the bitch.

The hormonal cycle of the queen is slightly different. As the queen is an induced ovulator, progesterone secreted by the corpus luteum will only be present if she is mated.

Behavioural changes and external signs

The bitch

Bitches usually have one or two oestrous cycles a year and during the period of oestrus they are described as being 'in season' or 'on heat'. The bitch is *monoestrous*, i.e. during each period of ovarian activity there is only one period of oestrus, and there is no recognised breeding season – bitches may come into season at any time of the year. The bitch is a *spontaneous ovulator*, i.e. ovulation occurs without the stimulus of mating and takes place around the tenth day of the cycle (Fig. 11.10).

Bitches reach sexual maturity or puberty at about 6 months but there is wide variation between breeds – larger breeds mature significantly later than smaller breeds. Puberty is marked by the onset of the first season. The phases of oestrous cycle are as follows:

- *Proestrus* – this lasts for about 9 days. The vulva becomes enlarged and there may be a blood-stained vaginal discharge. The bitch may urinate more frequently, which serves to advertise the fact that she is in season. She will be excitable and flirtatious with males and may try to escape to find them. However, if a male tries to mount her she will growl and clamp her tail tightly to her rump to prevent mating.

- *Oestrus* – this lasts for about 9 days. The vulva remains enlarged but the discharge becomes straw-coloured. The 'flirty' excitable behaviour continues and if a male dog attempts to mount her she will stand still, put her tail to one side and allow mating. *Ovulation* takes place on day 10 of the complete cycle (the first day of proestrus is counted as day 1) but there is no external sign.
- *Metoestrus* – this can be divided into two phases:
  - *Metoestrus I:* lasts for approximately 20 days, during which the vaginal discharge dries up, the swollen vulva shrinks and the bitch's behaviour returns to normal. At the end of this phase, the bitch appears to be back to normal, but internally the corpus luteum in the ovary continues to secrete progesterone.
  - *Metoestrus II:* lasts for approximately 70 days. There are no external signs, but the corpus luteum secretes progesterone, which causes the body to remain in an almost pregnancy-like state. In some bitches this causes overt symptoms of a *false pregnancy* or *pseudocyesis*.
- *Anoestrus* – this lasts for 3–9 months. The behaviour and appearance of the bitch are normal and there is almost no ovarian activity. Towards the end of this period, some of the primary follicles will begin to develop and secrete oestrogen and the cycle begins again.

The queen

The queen is *seasonally polyoestrus*. This means that she has several periods of oestrus or receptivity to the male during her breeding season, which is typically from January to September. Cats are 'long day breeders', stimulated to start cycling by the increasing hours of daylight that occur in the early spring. However, many domestic cats come into season all the year round as they live under the influence of central heating and electric light.

The queen is an *induced ovulator*, i.e. ovulation occurs in response to mating. The tip of the tomcat's penis is covered in tiny barbs which, when the penis is withdrawn at the end of mating, cause the queen a moment of pain. This starts a nerve pathway to the hypothalamus in the brain, and ultimately to the ovary, resulting in ovulation within 36 hours of mating.

Young queens become sexually mature in the spring after they are born. This means that if born in September, they may be as young as 4 months at the time of the first season in January/February. The phases of the oestrous cycle (Fig. 11.11) are as follows:

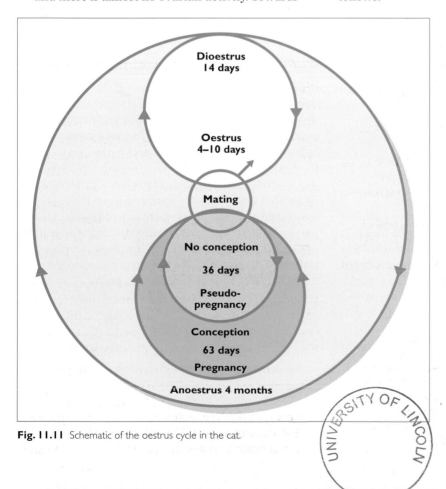

Fig. 11.11 Schematic of the oestrus cycle in the cat.

APPLIED ANATOMY

False pregnancies can occur in the cat but are very rare. If the queen is mated but does not conceive, a corpus luteum develops in the ovary and secretes progesterone which switches off further follicular development. After about 36 days, the corpus luteum regresses and the cycles start again. There are rarely any clinical signs associated with this phenomenon in cats.

- *Oestrus* – this lasts for 4–10 days but is very variable. There are no physical signs but the queen's behaviour includes rolling, rubbing against objects and *lordosis* (putting the rump in the air and the tail to one side). She will also 'call' – a loud persistent yowling sound–to inform all the tomcats in the area that she is receptive. If a tomcat approaches she will crouch down and allow mating to take place. As the queen is an induced ovulator, oestrus may continue until mating occurs. However, queens kept isolated from tomcats will eventually go into the next phase.
- *Dioetrus* – lasts for about 14 days. The queen's behaviour returns to normal and the ovary remains inactive for a short period. New follicles will begin to develop towards the end of this period and the cycle will begin again a few days later.
- *Anoestrus* – lasts for about 4 months and falls between September and January. During this period the ovary remains inactive and the queen is a 'normal' cat. As the day length increases, follicular development starts and the breeding season begins again.

EMBRYONIC AND FOETAL DEVELOPMENT

The *gestation period* is the interval between fertilisation of the ovum and the birth of the offspring. In the bitch and the queen, the gestation period is approximately 63 days, although there is both individual and breed variation. During gestation, complex changes occur to the zygote which result in a viable neonate nine weeks later.

Definitions

It is important to understand the terminology applied to the different stages of embryonic and foetal development.

- *Embryology* – the study of the development of the embryo
- *Gamete* – the male or female germ cells, i.e. spermatozoa (sperm) or ova
- *Zygote* – the fertilised ovum
- *Embryo* – the stage during which the major organs are forming
- *Fetus* – the stage at which formation of the major internal and external structures is complete until the time of parturition
- *Conceptus* – the embryo or fetus, the extra embryonic membranes and the placenta
- *Neonate* – a new-born animal.

Fertilisation and cell division

Each ovum released from the ovary during ovulation is covered in an outer protective layer of follicular cells known as the *corona radiata* and has an inner layer of glycoprotein known as the *zona pellucida*. The bitch and the queen are multiparous species, so they produce several ova at one time. The ova enter the infundibulum of the uterine tube and are transported down the uterine tube by muscular contractions and by the movements of the cilia of the epithelial lining.

After mating, sperm from the male travel up the female tract and fertilisation takes place within the upper part of the uterine tube. It is thought that sperm may live for as long as 7 days within the tract, relying on the correct environment within the uterine tube to survive. During this period the outer *acrosome* of the sperm (Fig. 11.4) releases enzymes which are able to break down the zona pellucida of the ovum. Each ovum is then penetrated by one sperm, which results in a *fertilisation reaction*, preventing fertilisation by any other sperm (Fig. 11.12). The fertilised ovum is now referred to as a *zygote* and cell division begins within a few hours of fertilisation.

Cell division occurs by *mitosis* (see Ch. 1): one cell divides into two, two into four, and so on. The stage in which the cells are too numerous to count is called a *morula*. A fluid-filled cavity develops inside the morula and the structure becomes a *blastocyst*. During this time the ball of cells is free-floating and moves slowly down the tract towards the uterine horns.

Implantation

Once in the uterine horns, the blastocysts arrange themselves at equal distances along the horns and may even cross from one horn to another to achieve equal spacing – a process known as *trans-uterine migration*. They then attach to the wall of the horns by

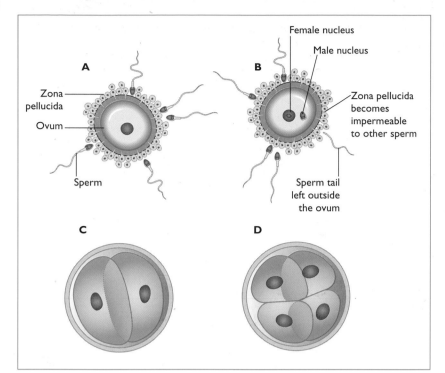

Fig. 11.12 Fertilisation of the ovum. **A** Spermatozoa approach ovum. **B** One sperm penetrates the ovum. **C, D** Cell division occurs by mitosis.

invading and partly destroying the hypertrophied endometrium, so that they are securely implanted. *Implantation* occurs between 14–20 days after ovulation in the bitch and 11–16 days after ovulation in the queen.

Development of the germ cell layers

Within the fluid-filled blastocyst, most of the cells come to lie on one side, forming the *inner cell mass*. A thinner layer of cells surrounding the fluid cavity form the *trophoblast* (Fig. 11.13). The inner cell mass becomes the embryo and, in the early stages, is a flat plate of cells. The trophoblast becomes the extra-embryonic membranes.

The cells now begin to form three *germ cell layers*, which eventually differentiate into parts of the embryo and the different membranes:

- The inner cell mass divides into:
  - An outer layer or *ectoderm* – forms the skin and nervous system
  - A middle layer or *mesoderm* – forms the musculoskeletal system and other internal organs
  - An inner layer or *endoderm* – forms the lining of the digestive tract and other visceral systems.
  Cells from the endoderm spread around to line the trophoblast and form the *yolk sac.* In mammals this

does not contain yolk, but in birds and reptiles the yolk sac is the source of nutrition for the embryo developing in the egg.

- The *trophoblast* lies around the outer part of the cavity (Fig 11.13). Between the yolk sac and the trophoblast, mesodermal cells split into two layers, between which is another cavity: one layer lies close to the trophoblast and later becomes the *chorion;* the other lies close to the endoderm/yolk sac.

The inner cell mass begins to curl around and enclose the endodermal and mesodermal cells, which form the internal organs, leaving the yolk sac and trophoblast to form the extra-embryonic membranes.

Development of the extra-embryonic membranes

The extra-embryonic membranes surround and protect the embryo but do not form the embryo itself:

- *Yolk sac* – formed from the endodermal cells, but shrivels to nothing some time before birth (Fig. 11.13).
- *Chorion* – formed from the trophoblast and the outer layer of mesodermal cells.
- *Amnion* – the trophoblast and mesoderm expand, and eventually push up and surround the developing embryo. This forms a fluid-filled cavity

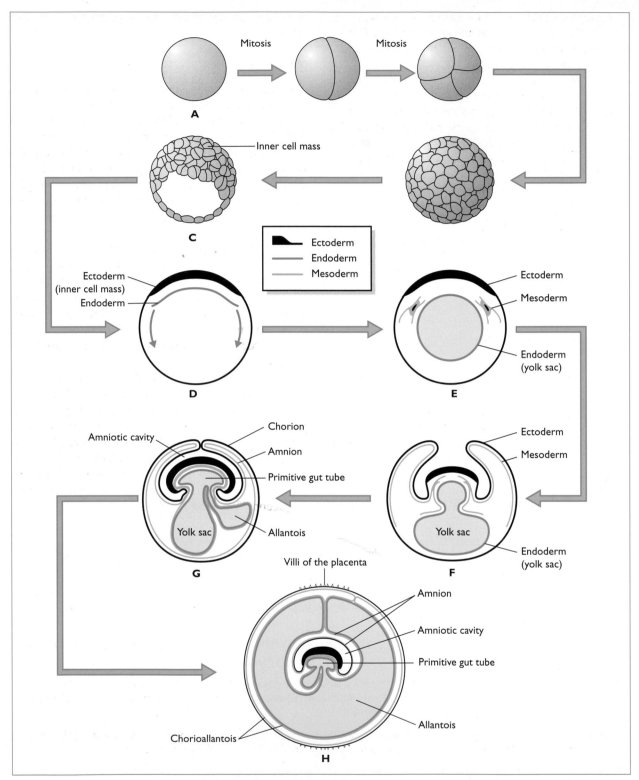

Fig. 11.13 Early embryonic development (see text also). **A** The fertilised cell divides by mitosis to form a ball of cells, the morula **(B)**. The morula develops a cavity and is known as the trophoblast **(C)**. A layer of endodermal cells starts to line the trophoblast **(D)** and forms the beginning of the yolk sac **(E)**. Blocks of mesoderm start to form as the inner cell mass starts to be pinched off to form the embryo mesoderm **(F)**. Another space forms from the primitive gut tube, this is the allantois **(G)** and the yolk sac begins to regress. Developing villi form a band around the extra-embryonic membranes **(H)**.

around the embryo – the *amniotic cavity* – which is entirely separate from all the other cavities. The outer layer is called the *amnion* and is the sac in which the fetus is delivered.

- *Allantois* – a balloon-like diverticulum starts to develop from the endodermal cells forming the primitive gut. It pushes out from the caudal end of the embryo and lies beside the yolk sac (Fig 11.13). This is the *allantois,* which collects urine from the foetal kidneys via a tube leading from the foetal bladder, the *urachus*. During development, the allantois continues to expand with foetal urine and eventually encircles the fetus. Its inner surface beomes part of the amnion, while its outer surface fuses with the chorion and becomes the *chorioallantois*. During parturition, the chorioallantois may be identified as the 'water bag', which ruptures to release the fetus within the amnion.

Development of the embryo

As the inner cell mass grows, the cells begin to curve underneath and the head and trunk are formed. Inside, the main body cavity or *coelom* is formed and later it is divided into thorax and abdomen by the diaphragm. All the internal organs are developed by 35 days – this process is known as *organogenesis*. After this, the fetus goes through a period of rapid growth until it reaches its final size prior to birth.

The later stages of development in a medium-sized breed of dog are summarised in Table 11.2. Kittens are often slightly in advance of puppies of the same stage.

The placenta

The placenta is a thickened vascular band which develops from the allantochorion around the centre of the conceptus. The allantochorion produces small finger-like villi which burrow into the endometrium of the uterine horn. Blood capillaries covering the membrane extend into the villi and come into close apposition with the blood capillaries of the endometrium. These form the maternal and foetal parts of the placenta, which are *not* continuous with each other.

The villi develop into broad bands running around the 'waist' of the conceptus. Nutrients and oxygen pass from the dam across the placenta and into the fetus via the umbilical blood vessels; waste products pass in the opposite direction. The *umbilical cord* contains the umbilical artery and vein, the remnants of the yolk sac and the stalk of the allantois connected to the urachus (see Ch. 7).

The placenta of the dog and cat is restricted to one zone and is therefore described as being a *zonary placenta*. Other species have more diffuse types of placenta. Between the placenta and the membranes, at the edge of the placenta, is an area where blood has escaped from broken blood capillaries and become trapped. This is the *marginal haematoma* and it stains the parturient discharges green in bitches and brown in queens. This discolouration is normal!

Table 11.2 The developmental stages of the canine embryo and fetus.	
Timescale	Stage of development
3 weeks	5 mm long; fore and hindlimbs are small buds sticking out from the trunk; amnion is complete and the allantois is formed
4 weeks	20 mm long; limbs are small cylinders with evidence of a paw shape; eyes are pigmented; external ear has a ridge of visible skin
5 weeks	35 mm long; ear flap is distinct; eyelids partly cover the eyes; digits can be seen on the paws; external genitalia are near to final positions; tactile (sinus) hairs are present on the upper lip; formation of internal organs (organogenesis) is complete
6 weeks	60 mm long; prominent scrotal or vulval tissues; digits widely spread; eyelids are fused; hair follicles and tactile follicles present on the body; claws present; ossification of skeleton at 45 days
7 weeks	100 mm long; body hair and colour markings are developing
8 weeks	150 mm long; hair covering is complete; pads have developed
9 weeks	Ready for birth

🔑 KEY POINTS

- The male gonad is the testis, responsible for spermatogenesis and the secretion of testosterone.

- The male reproductive tract conducts the sperm from the testis into the female reproductive tract during mating.

- The female gonad is the ovary, responsible for the production of ova and the secretion of oestrogen and progesterone.

- The release of ova from the ovary is associated with a regular cycle of interrelated hormonal changes in the ovary and the reproductive tract and in the animal's behavioural patterns – this is known as the oestrous cycle.

- Fertilisation occurs in the uterine tube and the developing embryos implant in the wall of the uterine horns.

- The extra-embryonic membranes and the embryo develop from different parts of the rapidly dividing ball of cells derived from the original fertilised ovum.

The term *common integument* refers to the outer covering of the body. It is said to be the largest organ of the body and, because it has a variety of component parts, it has a range of functions. The integument includes:

- Skin
- Hair
- Footpads
- Claws.

THE SKIN

The skin covers the external surface of the body, forming a complete barrier against the external environment. It is perforated by various natural openings, e.g. the mouth and the anus, and at these points it blends with the mucous membranes lining the openings. The functions of the skin are:

1. *Protection* – it protects the underlying structures of the body and in specialised thickened regions of the skin, e.g. pads of the feet, it gives added protection against physical trauma. It also acts as a physical barrier to protect against invasion by microorganisms and sebaceous glands secrete an antiseptic sebum onto the surface. The skin also acts as a water barrier as it is almost impermeable to water, preventing the body from drying out or from becoming waterlogged, e.g. when swimming. Pigmented areas in the skin and hair protect against damage from ultraviolet radiation.
2. *Sensory* – the surface of the skin is well supplied with many types of sensory nerve endings to detect temperature, pressure, touch and pain. This assists the body in monitoring its external environment.
3. *Secretion* – a range of glands within the skin produce secretions directly on to the skin's surface. These include *sebum* – produced by sebaceous glands; *sweat* – in the cat and dog sweating only occurs from active sweat glands of the footpads and nose; *pheromones* – produced by specialised skin glands.
4. *Production* – ultraviolet light from the sun converts 7-dihydrocholesterol present in sebum into vitamin D. This is activated within the kidney and liver and increases the uptake and metabolism of dietary calcium.

APPLIED ANATOMY

Dogs, cats and other species of animal that are kept indoors without access to sunlight may suffer from skeletal problems caused by the lack of vitamin D in their bodies. This is then reflected in the levels of calcium in the bones and tissues.

5. *Storage* – fat is stored under the skin as adipose tissue or subcutaneous fat. Fat is an energy store and also acts as a thermal insulating layer.
6. *Thermoregulation* – the skin prevents heat loss by diverting blood away from the surface by vasoconstriction, by erecting the hairs to trap a layer of insulating air, and by having an insulating layer of fat. Heat can be lost from the body when required, e.g. by the production of sweat. However, the skin only plays a minor role in heat loss in the dog and cat as they only have active sweat glands in their footpads and nose. Most of the dissipation of excessive body heat in dogs and cats occurs via panting.
7. *Communication* – production of pheromones, which are natural scents used for intraspecific communication. Other 'scents' produced for communication are those of the circumanal glands and glands of the anal sacs. The integument also provides a means of visual communication, e.g. a dog raises its hackles when threatened, which is seen as a warning of possible aggression.

Skin structure

The skin is composed of two layers: the *epidermis* or superficial layer and the underlying *dermis* (Fig. 12.1). The *hypodermis* lies beneath the skin.

Epidermis

The epidermis is composed of *stratified squamous epithelium* and has multiple layers of cells that are continually renewed. New cells are produced in the deepest layers of the epidermis and are pushed upwards to the surface as a result of mitosis below (see Ch. 1). The surface cells are continually lost and these dead cells or *squames* are seen as scurf in the animal's coat. This process replaces the cells that are lost due to friction and wear. The layers, or *strata*, of the epidermis are, from deep to superficial:

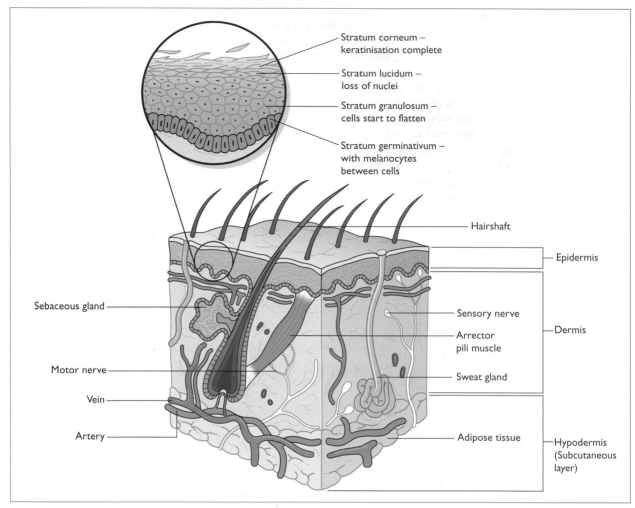

Stratum corneum –
keratinisation complete

Stratum lucidum –
loss of nuclei

Stratum granulosum –
cells start to flatten

Stratum germinativum –
with melanocytes
between cells

Hairshaft

Epidermis

Sebaceous gland

Sensory nerve

Arrector
pili muscle

Dermis

Motor nerve

Sweat gland

Vein

Artery

Adipose tissue

Hypodermis
(Subcutaneous
layer)

Fig. 12.1 Structure of the skin.

APPLIED ANATOMY

The colour of the skin and overlying hair may not necessarily be the same and this may be noticed when clipping an area for a surgical operation. It is interesting to note that the skin of polar bears is black but the fur is white!

1. *Stratum basale* or *germinativum* – consists of a single layer of dividing cells, i.e. where the new cells are 'manufactured'. Pigmented cells or *melanocytes,* which contain granules of the pigment melanin, may also be present in areas such as the nose pad or footpad or in coloured areas of the body.
2. *Stratum granulosum* – the cells are flattened and the process of infiltration of the cells by the structural protein *keratin* (known as *keratinisation*) begins in this layer. Keratin provides protection in layers that get extra wear, e.g. footpads.
3. *Stratum lucidum* – the cells lose their nuclei and become clearer.

4. *Stratum corneum* – the most superficial of the epidermal layers. The cells have no nuclei and are dead; they are fully keratinised and flattened in shape.

The whole of the epidermis is avascular and receives its supply of nutrients from blood vessels within the dermis.

Dermis

The dermis is the deep layer of the skin, upon which the epidermis sits (Fig. 12.1). It is composed of dense connective tissue with irregularly arranged collagen and elastic fibres. The dermis has a generous supply of blood vessels, nerves and sensory nerve endings. The hair follicles, sebaceous glands and sweat glands also lie within the dermis but are formed from epidermal cells.

Hypodermis

The hypodermis, or subcutis or subcuticular layer, is not actually part of the skin, but is a layer of loose connective tissue and fat lying beneath the dermis. It also contains elastic fibres, which gives the skin its flexibility. This is evident when we grasp a fold of skin on the neck of a dog or cat to 'scruff' them. It is the hypodermis into which subcutaneous injections are given.

Skin glands

Within the dermis are a range of glands producing secretions directly on to the skin surface:

Sebaceous glands

These are alveolar or saccular glands whose ducts open into the base of the hair follicles. They secrete an oily substance called *sebum* which forms a waterproof layer on the skin and coat, giving the coats 'sheen' and making the skin supple. It has an antiseptic quality which controls bacterial growth on the skin surface. Some of the modified sebaceous glands produce secretions that influence the behaviour of another animal. These are known as pheromones and are the 'scents' that dogs and cats produce as a means of communicating between members of their own species.

Modified sebaceous glands include:

■ *Tail glands* – these are found on the dorsal surface of the base of the tail. Their function is believed to be concerned with individual recognition and identification.
■ *Circumanal glands* – these are located around the entire circumference of the anus. They drain into special sweat glands and their secretion is thought to contribute to the individual smell of a dog.
■ *Anal glands* – these lie within the walls of the paired spherical anal sacs, located on either side and just below the anus. They produce a foul smelling secretion that is expressed during defecation, coating the faeces and serving as a territorial marker.
■ *Circumoral glands* – these glands are found on the lips of cats and their secretion is used for territorial marking. This can be observed when a cat rubs its face on objects such as furniture and its owner's legs!
■ *Ceruminous glands* – found in the external ear canal, they secrete cerumen or ear wax.
■ *Meibomian* or *tarsal glands* – these open onto the eyelids and produce the fatty component of the tear film that moistens the eye.

Sweat glands

Also called *sudoriferous* glands. These are coiled glands found in the dermis which are only active on the nose and footpads of dogs and cats.

Mammary glands

These are greatly modified, enlarged sweat glands, which secrete milk for nourishment of the young (see Ch. 11).

APPLIED ANATOMY

In areas of the body that are covered in hair, the epidermis of the skin may only be a few cells thick, e.g. the skin over the abdomen. However in areas unprotected by hair, e.g. the footpads, the epidermis is much thicker. This can easily be seen when examining a cut pad.

HAIR

The possession of hair or fur is a distinctive characteristic of mammals. It covers the entire body of the dog and cat except in areas such as the nose and footpads. In other areas, such as the scrotum and around the nipples, the hair covering is much sparser.

A hair is a keratinised structure and is produced by a *hair follicle*. The visible part of the hair, above the skin's surface, is called the *hair shaft* and the part of the hair that lies within the follicle is called the *hair root*.

The hair follicle originates from a peg of epidermal cells which grows down into the underlying dermis, where it forms a *hair cone* over a piece of dermis called the *dermal papilla* (Fig. 12.2). The papilla provides the blood and nerve supply for the growing hair. From the hair cone, the cells keratinise and form a hair. As the hair grows up through the epidermis to the skin's surface, the cells at the point of the cone die, forming a channel – the hair follicle. The hair continues to grow until it eventually dies and becomes detached from the follicle. Hair growth is cyclical and once the hair is shed a new hair follicle develops and a new hair will start to grow.

Moulting

The shedding of hair or *moulting* is influenced by the annual seasons, particularly the environmental temperature and day length. Most dogs moult more heavily in the spring and autumn, while cats only moult heavily in spring followed by a lighter loss of hair throughout the summer and autumn. However, pet cats and dogs are usually kept inside centrally heated houses with electric lighting and this confuses the natural seasonal triggers. Moulting can therefore occur to some extent all year round.

Hair types

There are three major types of hair:

1. *Guard hairs* – these are the thick, long and stiff hairs that form the outer protective coat of the animal. They lie closely against the skin and sweep uniformly in broad tracts giving the coat of a dog or cat its smooth appearance. The nature of

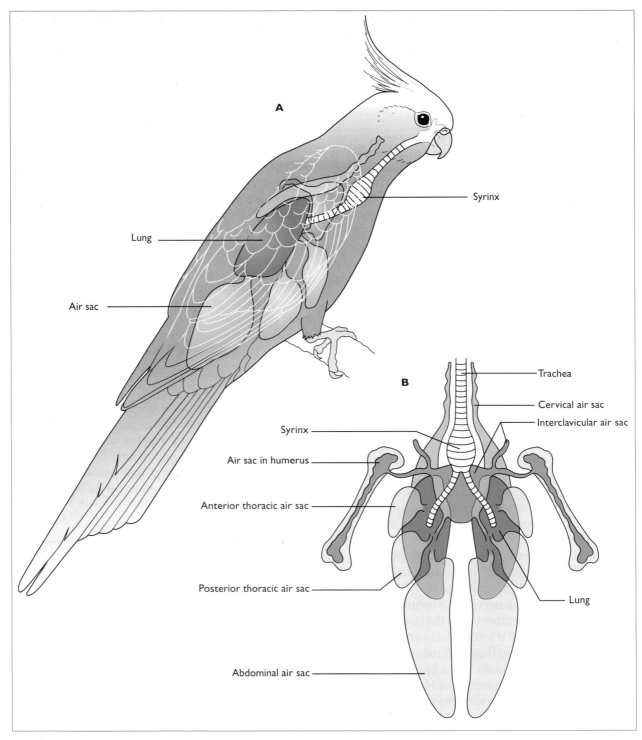

Fig. 13.9 The respiratory system of the bird in situ **(A)** and removed from the body **(B)**.

APPLIED ANATOMY

Some diving birds do not have external nares as this would allow water to enter the airways during diving. They normally rely on mouth breathing. If the beak is tied to prevent the bird from pecking during treatment, there is a risk of asphyxiation.

Air passes through the *glottis* on the floor of the oral cavity and into a complex *larynx*. It travels down the *trachea* to the point where the trachea divides into right and left primary *bronchi*. At this point there is a swelling known as the *syrinx*, whose size and shape varies with the species. The combined effect of air passing through the larynx and the syrinx produces the characteristic sounds associated with the species.

APPLIED ANATOMY

Birds are easily intubated for anaesthesia as the glottis at the base of the tongue is easy to see. Always use an *uncuffed tube* to prevent rupture of the incomplete tracheal rings. The caudal air sacs may also be intubated after induction by injection or by mask, in cases where oral or beak surgery is to be performed.

The primary bronchi lead into the relatively dense lungs, closely applied to the dorsal body wall. Within the lung tissue the bronchi divide into further smaller bronchi and into cylindrical parallel tubes known as *parabronchi*. Air capillaries surrounded by pulmonary blood capillaries perforate the walls of the parabronchi and it is here that gaseous exchange takes place. This process is the same as occurs in mammals.

Leading from various bronchi within the lungs are thin-walled *air sacs*. Most birds have nine air sacs, which penetrate the spaces of the body cavity and the inside of many bones (Fig. 13.9). They are not involved in gaseous exchange and they are thought to act as a reservoir of air and to have a bellows-effect, pushing air back through the lungs. They also lighten the weight of the skeleton and so aid flight.

Respiration (Fig. 13.10)

During respiration air circulates continuously and passes through the lungs twice. Most gaseous exchange occurs during the second passage. This system ensures that the removal of oxygen from the inspired air occurs with maximum efficiency.

■ *Inspiration* – air passes through the lungs and either enters:

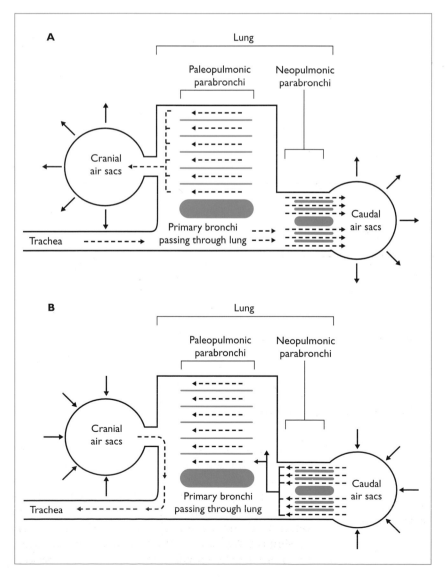

Fig. 13.10 Diagram to show the passage of air through the lungs and air sacs during respiration. **A** Inspiration. **B** Expiration.

- The caudal air sacs and inflates them, or
- The parabronchi, where gaseous exchange takes place; this air then passes into the cranial air sacs and inflates them.

■ *Expiration*
  - The abdominal muscles contract, squeezing air from the caudal air sacs back into the parabronchi, where further gaseous exchange takes place
  - Air in the cranial air sacs passes straight through the lungs and out.

CIRCULATORY SYSTEM

The circulatory system follows a similar plan to that of the mammal. In order to provide for the high metabolic rate of the bird, the heart in particular must be able to pump the blood to deliver oxygen and nutrients to the tissues quickly and efficiently. In a resting chicken blood takes only six seconds to travel around the body.

Main features

Heart

This is a four-chambered pump lying in the cranial part of the thoracoabdominal cavity. It is covered in a pericardial sac which sticks to some of the internal surfaces to hold the heart in place.

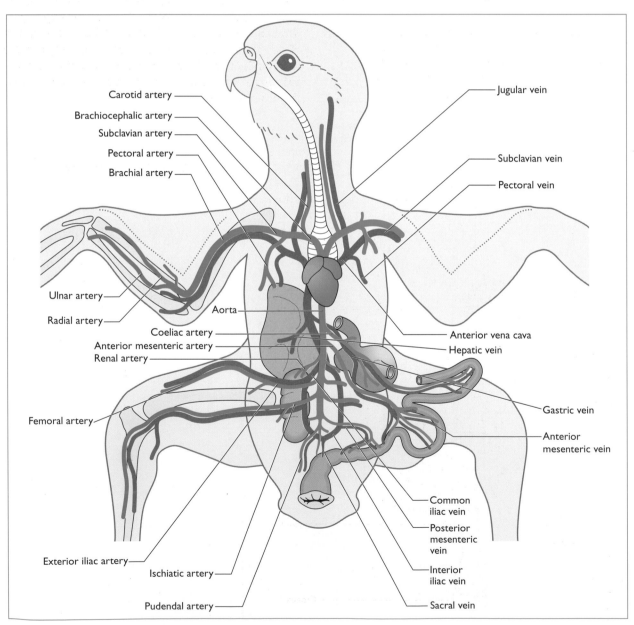

Carotid artery
Brachiocephalic artery
Subclavian artery
Pectoral artery
Brachial artery

Jugular vein

Subclavian vein

Pectoral vein

Ulnar artery
Radial artery
Aorta
Coeliac artery
Anterior mesenteric artery
Renal artery

Anterior vena cava
Hepatic vein

Femoral artery

Gastric vein

Anterior mesenteric vein

Common iliac vein
Posterior mesenteric vein
Interior iliac vein

Exterior iliac artery
Ischiatic artery
Pudendal artery

Sacral vein

Fig. 13.11 The avian circulatory system.

Circulation (Fig. 13.11)

The arrangement of the arteries, veins and capillaries is similar to that of mammals with the following differences:

- *Renal portal system* – valves at the junction of the iliac veins with the caudal vena cava can divert blood returning from the caudal end of the body either into the kidneys, so excreting waste products, or into the caudal vena cava and so to the heart.
- There is a large blood supply to the flight muscles and wings via the *pectoral* and *brachial arteries*.
- Heat loss from the legs and feet of many terrestrial and aquatic species is reduced by a counter-current system of blood vessels in the lower limbs.

APPLIED ANATOMY

Intravenous injections or blood sampling can be carried out using the brachial vein on the medial side of the wing close to the elbow joint, the jugular vein in the neck and the medial metatarsal vein on the caudal aspect of the leg.

Body heat in the arteries of the limbs is transferred to the blood returning to the heart in the veins, which lie parallel to the arteries. This means that the legs and feet are kept cool, reducing the temperature gradient between the blood and the external air, so less heat is lost from areas which are not insulated by feathers.

Blood

The erythrocytes or red blood cells are oval and nucleated which is different from those of mammals but similar to those of reptiles.

DIGESTIVE SYSTEM

The basic pattern of the digestive tract is much the same between species of birds and the upper part shows adaptations for flight (Fig. 13.12). The majority of the tract is suspended between the wings in the body cavity to centralise the weight, enabling the bird to keep its balance and remain stable in flight without the use of a long tail.

Fig. 13.12 Digestive system of the pigeon.

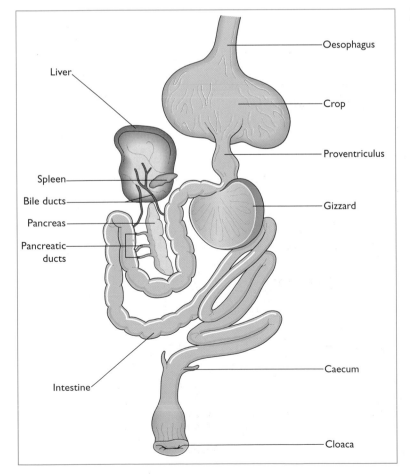

Labels: Liver, Spleen, Bile ducts, Pancreas, Pancreatic ducts, Intestine, Oesophagus, Crop, Proventriculus, Gizzard, Caecum, Cloaca

Main features

Oral cavity

The teeth, heavy jaw bones and muscles have been replaced by a beak and lighter bones and muscles. Birds are unable to chew their food but can manipulate it and break it into small pieces using the *beak* and the *tongue.* The shape of the beak varies according to species and is suited to the particular food type (Fig. 13.13). *Salivary glands* are present in most species and the saliva contains mucus. In some species, such as the sparrows, the saliva is also rich in the enzyme amylase. *Taste buds* are found towards the back of the oral cavity and their structure is similar to those in other species.

Oesophagus and crop (Fig. 13.12)

Food passes down the oesophagus on the right side of the neck into the *crop.* The oesophagus is thin-walled and distensible to allow the passage of relatively large pieces of food. The crop is a diverticulum of the oesophagus, lying outside the body cavity on the right side of the cranial thoracic inlet. It varies in size and shape according to the diet of the species – grain-eating birds have large bilobed crops while in owls and insectivores the crop may be rudimentary or absent.

The crop is principally a storage organ but in some species, e.g. doves and pigeons, the epithelial lining proliferates and sloughs under the influence of the hormone prolactin to produce 'crop milk'. This is rich in proteins and fat and is used to feed the young for the first few days after hatching.

Stomach

Food passes into the stomach, which has two parts:

1. *Proventriculus* – lined by gastric glands which secrete pepsin, hydrochloric acid and mucus. Here food is stored and mixed with these digestive juices.
2. *Gizzard (ventriculus)* – thick-walled muscular organ in which mechanical digestion occurs. By means of powerful contractions the food is ground up and mixed with the digestive juices. The presence of grit in the diet helps the physical break up of the food. In species which feed on softer or liquid foods the gizzard is mainly a storage organ

Small intestine

Food leaves the gizzard by the pylorus and enters the small intestine, which consists of a duodenum and ileum (Fig. 13.12). Beyond this there is no clear delineation into different parts. The pancreas, consisting of three lobes, lies in the duodenal loop and pours its secretions into the duodenum via three ducts. The liver is bilobed and relatively large and some species, e.g. chickens, ducks and geese, have a gallbladder.

Large intestine

This consists of a pair of blind-ending *caecae,* originating at the junction of the small and large intestines, a

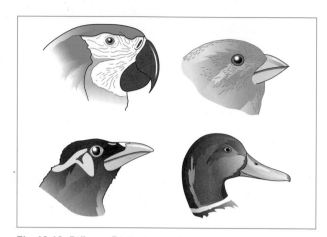

Fig. 13.13 Differences in beak shape between species.

rectum and a *cloaca.* Bacterial digestion occurs in the caecae which are large and prominent in herbivorous and granivorous species and owls, but are rudimentary or absent in carnivorous and nectivorous species, e.g. hawks and parrots.

The rectum is short and terminates at the cloaca – the common exit from the body cavity shared with the urinary and reproductive systems.

URINARY SYSTEM

This consists of a pair of symmetrical kidneys lying in a depression of the fused pelvic bones (Figs 13.14 and 13.15). A pair of ureters carries urine to the outside via the cloaca. There is no bladder in the bird. The kidneys are relatively larger than those of mammals and occupy about 2% of body weight.

Birds excrete nitrogenous waste resulting from protein metabolism in the form of uric acid and urates. This is similar to reptiles but different from mammals, which excrete nitrogenous waste as urea. The waste materials are suspended in urinary water resulting from glomerular filtration and the resulting semi-solid urine leaves the kidneys via the ureters. In the cloaca it mixes with faecal material from the digestive tract. The material then moves by retroperistalsis into the rectum where further reabsorption of water takes place, eventually producing a small volume of 'droppings'. Normal bird droppings (Fig. 13.16) consist of white urates and greeny-brown faeces surrounded by clear urine.

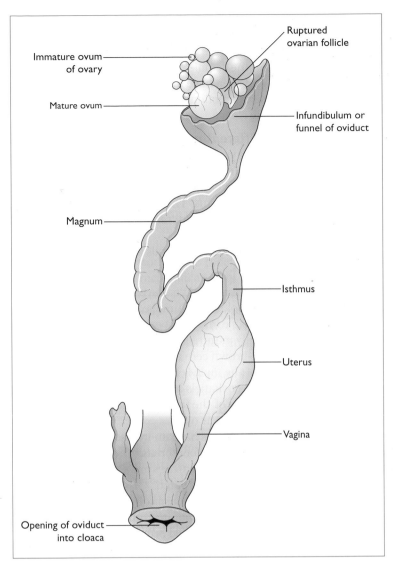

Fig. 13.14 Reproductive tract of the hen.

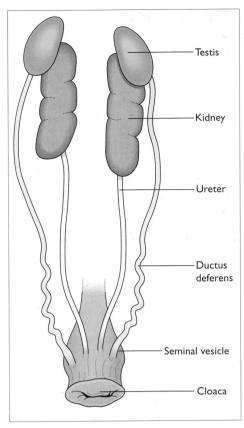

Fig. 13.15 Urogenital system of the male bird.

APPLIED ANATOMY

Many species of marine bird have a *salt gland* that enables them to deal with a salt water environment. In most birds it is located above the eye and secretes large quantities of sodium chloride. In this way the osmotic concentration of the body fluids is maintained within normal limits. Terrestrial species rely on the kidneys to regulate salt levels.

REPRODUCTIVE SYSTEM

Female (Fig. 13.14)

The tract comprises a pair of ovaries and oviducts leading to the cloaca. However, in many species it is only the left side that it is fully developed and functional, the right side being vestigial. Ova develop within the ovarian tissue and consist of an oocyte and a yolk surrounded by several layers of cells. During the breeding season one ovum is released at approximately 24 hour intervals until the clutch is complete.

Domestic poultry have been selectively bred to lay eggs over long periods – usually for 40 weeks per year. Wild birds will lay a clutch of eggs of a size appropriate to their species and then begin incubation.

The ovum is carried away down the left oviduct by peristaltic contractions. The oviduct is divided into distinct regions, each one of which contributes to the final egg:

1. *Infundibulum* – the funnel-shaped end of the oviduct which engulfs the ovum, preventing it from falling into the body cavity. Fertilisation takes place here and the first layer of albumen is added.

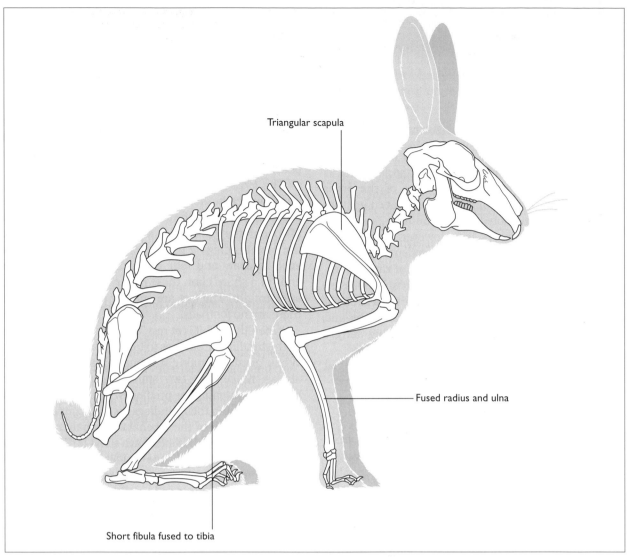

Triangular scapula

Fused radius and ulna

Short fibula fused to tibia

Fig. 14.1 Skeleton of the rabbit showing main features.

- The *acetabulum* or socket of the hip joint comprises the ilium, ischium and an accessory bone, the os acetabuli. The pubis is not involved in the formation of this socket, as is seen in the cat.
- In the *forelimb* the radius and ulna are completely fused; in the cat they are separate bones.
- In the *hindlimb* the fibula is half the length of the tibia and is fused with it; in the cat they are separate bones.
- Rabbit muscle is also a much paler pink than the muscle of cats.

Digestive system

Rabbits are herbivorous and have been likened to 'little horses' in that both the rabbit and the horse are hind gut fermenters, i.e. the main chamber for the breakdown of plant material is part of the large intestine. Unlike the horse, however, the digestive system of the rabbit allows for rapid passage of food through the tract and rapid elimination of fibre. This has enabled the body size and weight of the rabbit to remain small, which allows the animal to show the speed and agility necessary to escape predators. By contrast, in the horse, fibre remains in the gut for some time, necessitating the evolution of a large-volumed fermentation chamber and consequently a large body size. The digestive tract of the rabbit (Fig. 14.3) is relatively long and makes up 10–20% of body weight.

Oral cavity

The opening of the mouth is small, the tongue is relatively large and the oral cavity is long and curved, making examination of the cheek teeth and intubation for anaesthesia difficult. All the teeth (Fig. 14.4) are open rooted and grow continuously throughout life. They must be kept worn down by hard or fibrous food materials. The dental formula is:

$$[I2/1, C0/0, PM3/2, M3/3] \times 2 = 28 \text{ total.}$$

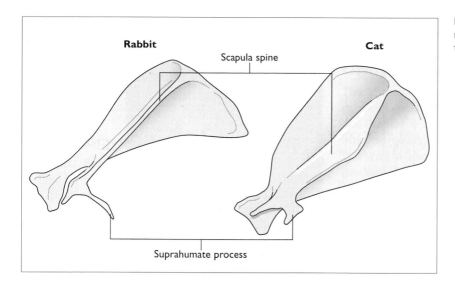

Fig. 14.2 The scapula of the rabbit compared to that of that cat.

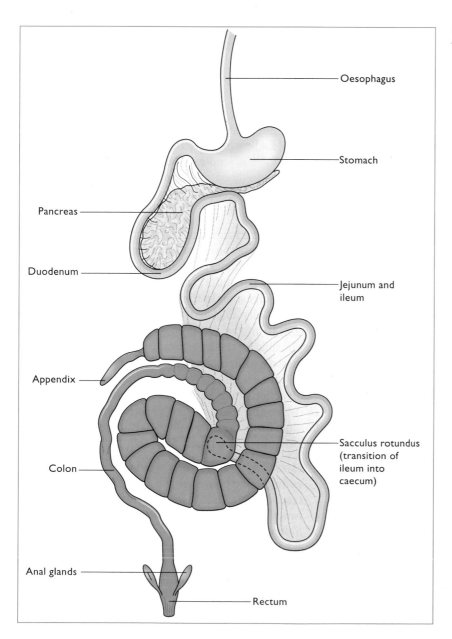

Fig. 14.3 Digestive system of the rabbit.

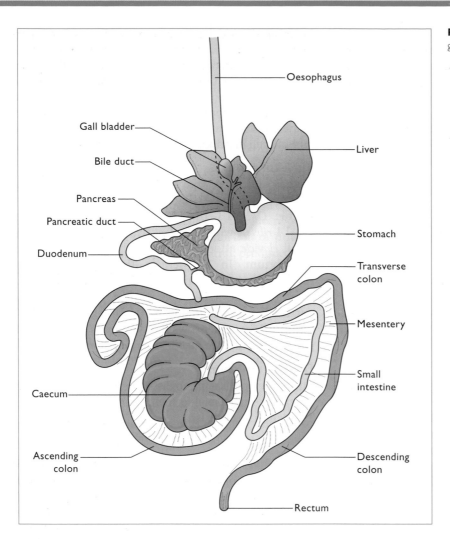

Fig. 14.10 The digestive system of the guinea pig.

The *oral cavity* is small and narrow and contains the relatively large *tongue*. There are four pairs of *salivary glands* which empty into the oral cavity near the molars. The *soft palate* is continuous with the base of the tongue and the *oropharynx* connects with the rest of the *pharynx* via a hole in the soft palate known as the *palatal ostium*.

The *stomach* (Fig. 14.10) is simple and is lined by a glandular epithelium. Gastric emptying takes about two hours. The intestinal tract measures approximately 2 m. The *small intestine* lies mainly on the right side of the abdominal cavity while the much longer *large intestine* fills the central and left parts of the abdomen. The most significant organ is the *caecum*, measuring 15–20 cm, and which is thin walled and sacculated with many lateral pouches created by thick bands of smooth muscle. At any one time it may contain 65% of the gut contents. The caecum contains microorganisms which are responsible for the breakdown of cellulose in the plant cell walls and for the addition of certain nutrients such as vitamin B.

The total time taken for food to pass through the digestive tract is approximately 20 hours but may take as long as 66 hours if coprophagia is taken into account. Guinea pigs exhibit *coprophagia* or *caecotrophy* and may be seen to eat softer more mucoid caecotrophs direct from the anus between 150–200 times a day. The liver has six lobes and there is a well-developed gall bladder.

APPLIED ANATOMY

When attempting to pass a feeding tube through the palatal ostium into the oesophagus, make sure it does not slip to one side and damage the surrounding vascular soft palate.

APPLIED ANATOMY

The liver of the guinea pig is unable to synthesise vitamin C and deficiencies may occur if the animal does not receive a daily dietary source. Symptoms include a dull rough coat, stiff gait and lameness, pain on movement, diarrhoea, anorexia and general lethargy.

Urinary system

Each *kidney* has a relatively large renal pelvis with a single papilla. The *urine* produced by the guinea pig is alkaline, thick and often a cloudy white or yellow. The presence of crystals in urine is a normal finding.

Reproductive system

- *Male* – known as a *boar*. The two *testes* are able to pass through the inguinal canal, which remains open throughout life. In mature breeding boars the large testes lie in the scrotum on either side of the genital opening. Internally there are several *accessory glands* – the long coiled vesicular glands, prostate, coagulating glands and the bulbourethral glands. There is an *os penis* and caudoventral to the urethral opening is a pouch containing two horny *styles* or projections which evert externally during erection of the penis.
- *Female* – known as a *sow*. The uterus is *bicornuate* and consists of two long uterine horns, a short body and a cervix leading into the vagina.

The female guinea pig is *polyoestrous* and a *spontaneous ovulator*. Details can be found in Table 14.2 (p 189). The gestation period is 63 days, which is long compared to that of other rodents, and the young are *precocial*, i.e. they are born fully furred with their eyes open and can be independent of their mothers. This enables them to eat solid food, although for the first few weeks they also suckle from the mother. They are born in the open, unprotected by a nest, and have to move around and escape predators if necessary.

Sexual differentiation

Guinea pigs are easy to sex and this can be done almost from birth.

- *Male* – mature boars have clearly defined testes. The penis can be prolapsed by applying gentle pressure at its base, cranial to the urethral opening.
- *Female* – the perineal tissues form a Y-shaped depression. The vulval opening lies at the intersection of the Y, with the anus at the base of the Y. If pressure is applied cranial to the vulval opening, there will be no penile prolapse.

Both sexes of guinea pig have a pair of inguinal nipples

Chinchilla (*Chinchilla lanigera*)

Morphology

Chinchillas originate in the mountains of South America and were imported into the United Kingdom for the fur trade. Nowadays, with a change in attitude towards the wearing of fur, chinchillas are mainly kept as pets. They are almost extinct in the wild and the only species likely to be found in captivity is C. *lanigera*. Chinchillas have a compact body with short limbs and a short bushy tail. They weigh from 400–500 g and the females are larger than the males. The nose is pointed and there are long sensitive whiskers on the divided upper lip. They have dark, prominent eyes on either side of the head which are adapted to seeing in poor light and they have large, round, delicate ears. At rest the chinchilla sits upright supported by its large hindfeet and uses its forepaws for holding food. They have four clawed toes on each fore and hind paw and the palmar and plantar surfaces of the feet are hairless.

The natural colour of the fur is blue-grey. The fur is soft and very dense which is due to the fact that as many as 60 hairs may grow from a single follicle. When fluffed up, the chinchilla appears to be deceptively large but under the fur the skeleton is quite small. Selective breeding has produced a range of other colours.

Digestive system

Like the guinea pig, chinchillas are *monogastric herbivores* with a large caecum for the breakdown of cellulose. The dental formula is:

$$[I1/1, C0/0, PM1/1, M3/3] \times 2 = 20 \text{ total}.$$

Teeth are present in the jaw at birth. Both the *incisors* and the cheek teeth (*premolars* and *molars*) are open rooted and grow continuously throughout the chinchilla's life. The chisel-shaped incisors, which are yellower than those of the guinea pig, have been reported as growing as much as 6 cm in a year. The cheek teeth are flattened table teeth for grinding fibrous plant material. The space between the incisors and the cheek teeth is known as the *diastema*. As with all species of rodent, dental problems are one of the most common conditions seen by veterinary surgeons.

The *oral cavity* is small and narrow. Like guinea pigs, the base of the tongue is continuous with the soft palate and the entrance to the pharynx is via a small hole, the *palatal ostium*.

The stomach is relatively large and simple. The intestine is long and has evolved to digest plant material. The caecum is long and coiled and holds a smaller percentage of the total intestinal contents than in the guinea pig or rabbit. The colon is sacculated. Microbial fermentation occurs within the caecum, resulting in the formation of caecotrophs which are rich in nutrients such as vitamin B. The chinchilla exhibits coprophagia but digestive studies show that while the guinea pig ingests both caecotrophs and faecal pellets at intervals throughout the day, the chinchilla only consumes faecal pellets at night and caecotrophs between 8am and 2pm.

APPLIED ANATOMY

The chinchilla has evolved to survive on the relatively poor but highly fibrous diet of grasses found high up in the Andes. A healthy diet for a chinchilla should therefore include high levels of fibre and protein. Treats such as apples, figs and sultanas must be given in moderation. It is not uncommon for chinchillas to die from constipation or diarrhoea caused by an over indulgent owner.

Reproductive system

■ *Male* – there is no true scrotum. The *testes* remain in the open inguinal canal or in the abdomen. On either side of the anus are two *postanal sacs* in which the caudal epididymis can lie. In the presence of a female the testes swell and become very obvious. The *penis,* which may be 1.5 cm long in the adult, is easily visible below the anus, from which it is separated by a small area of hairless skin. It is supported by the presence of a small bone known as the *baculum.*

■ *Female* – the uterus consists of two long *uterine horns,* each of which terminates in a *cervix.* This is similar to the rabbit but different from the structure seen in the guinea pig. The two cervices then lead into the single *vagina.* Both male and female chinchillas have three pairs of *mammary glands* – one inguinal pair and two lateral thoracic ones. The teats tend to protrude sideways, allowing the young to sit beside the dam and suckle.

The female chinchilla is *seasonally polyoestrous* and a *spontaneous ovulator.* Details can be found in Table 14.2 (p 189). The gestation period is 111 days, which is exceptionally long for a member of the rodent family. The young are *precocial,* i.e. they are born fully furred and capable of living an independent life. However, they continue to suckle from the dam until they are weaned at about 6–8 weeks.

Sexual differentiation

Chinchillas are quite easy to sex and this can be done at birth.

■ *Male* – as with many rodent species, the anogenital distance is longer in the male than it is in the female (Fig. 14.7). The penis can be extruded by gentle pressure at its base.

■ *Female* – the anogenital distance is shorter. A relatively large urinary papilla lies close to the anus and can be mistaken for a penis; however, there is no hairless band between it and the anus. The opening to the urethra is on the tip of this papilla and the opening to the slit-like vulva is immediately caudal to it.

THE FERRET

The domestic ferret, *Mustela putorius furo,* is a member of the order Carnivora and the family Mustelidae. Other related species include badgers, otters, stoats and weasels, all of which are long bodied agile creatures capable of producing a characteristic pungent smell from their anal glands.

Ferrets are most closely related to the European polecat, *Mustela putorius,* found in parts of the United Kingdom and northern Europe. It is almost certain that the Egyptians domesticated the polecat to produce the modern ferret. Although working ferrets are still used for hunting rabbits and rats, nowadays ferrets are becoming more popular as pets and in the USA there may be as many as 7 million pet ferrets!

Morphology

The ferret has a flexible tubular body with short legs and a long thick tail. This shape enables it to go down rabbit holes and to squeeze through openings in a cage or in the house – so steps must be taken to prevent escape! The *neck* is long and muscular and of the approximately the same diameter as the rest of the body. The *head* is relatively small with small ears set wide apart on the crown. The eyes point forward and are also set wide apart, providing binocular vision. However, ferrets' eyesight is poor and adapted to the low light levels found in tunnels.

The *legs* are short and used for digging and traction, but the ferret is also able to climb and may scale great heights. There are five toes on each *foot,* ending in non-retractable claws; in working ferrets these are kept long. The first digit on each foot has only two phalanges while the remainder have three.

The *skin* of the ferret is thick, especially over the neck and shoulders where it provides protection against bites. It is well supplied with *sebaceous glands* which are the main source of the ferret's body odour.

Ferrets also have a pair of well developed *anal glands* which produce a yellow serous secretion with a strong smell. The *fur* is thick and in the past this has led to ferrets being used in the fur trade. The natural colour is a cream undercoat with black guard hairs, black feet and tail and a black mask on the face. This is the colouration of the polecat and in the ferret is known as 'fitch'. Other naturally occurring colours are albino and sandy or cinnamon. Selective breeding of pet ferrets has led to the development of about 30 other colour variations. Ferrets moult in the spring and autumn and the fur may vary between the seasons: it may be shorter and darker in the summer months and longer and lighter in the winter.

Musculoskeletal system

The general pattern of the skeleton is shown in Figures 14.11 and 14.12. The vertebral formula is C7, T15, L5–6, S3, Cd18. The spine is extremely flexible and allows the ferret to bend at an angle of at least 180°. Ribs 1–10 attach to the sternum and the remainder form the costal arch. The thoracic inlet is very small and the presence of any abnormal mass here may interfere with swallowing and respiration.

Digestive system

The ferret is a true carnivore and this is reflected in the anatomy of its dentition and digestive tract (Fig. 14.13). As in other carnivores, the teeth are very sharp and adapted for shearing flesh off bone. The dental formula is:

$$[I3/3, C1/1, PM3/3, M1/2] \times 2 = 34 \text{ total.}$$

The *incisors* are prominent, the upper incisors being slightly longer and covering the lower ones. The *canines* are large and the roots are longer than the crown – they may be visible when the mouth is closed. The third upper premolars are the largest cheek teeth and are known as the *carnassials*. The deciduous teeth erupt at 20–28 days and the permanent teeth at 50–74 days.

In common with other carnivores, the length of the digestive tract (Fig. 14.11) is short; this results in a short gastrointestinal transit time of 3–4 hours in the adult animal. The *stomach* is simple and small, but capable of enormous distension to hold a large amount of food prior to its digestion. The pylorus is well developed. The stomach lies within a curve of the six-lobed *liver* in the anterior abdomen. The ferret has a pear-shaped *gall bladder* and its *pancreas* has two

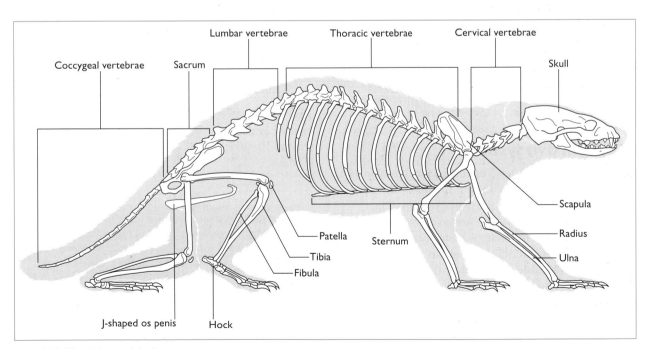

Fig. 14.11 The skeleton of the ferret.

Table 14.1 Physiological and behavioural parameters of rabbits and small rodents.

	Rabbit	Chinchilla	Chipmunk	Gerbil	Guinea pig	Golden hamster	Mouse	Rat
Average lifespan	6–8 years	10 years	2–6 years	3–5 years	4–8 years	2–3 years	2–3 years	3–4 years
Adult weight	1–8 kg	400–600 g	70–120 g	50–60 g	750–1000 g	100 g	20–40 g	400–800 g
Body temp. (°C)	38.3	38.0–39.0	38.0	37.4–39.0	38.6	36.2–37.5	37.5	38.0
Respiratory rate	35–60/min	40–80/min	70/min	90–140/min	90–150/min	74/min	100–250/min	70–150/min
Pulse rate	220/min	100–150/min	120/min	250–500/min	130–190/min	280–412/min	500–600/min	260–450/min
Dietary habits	Herbivorous; coprophagic	Herbivorous; coprophagic	Omnivorous; coprophagic	Omnivorous; coprophagic	Herbivorous; needs Vit. C; coprophagic	Omnivorous; coprophagic	Omnivorous; coprophagic	Omnivorous; coprophagic
Natural behaviour	Social; crepuscular	Social; nocturnal	Social; diurnal	Social; nocturnal	Social; diurnal	Solitary; nocturnal	Social; nocturnal	Social; nocturnal

Table 14.2 Reproductive data relating to rabbits and small rodents.

	Rabbit	Chinchilla	Chipmunk	Gerbil	Guinea pig	Golden hamster	Mouse	Rat
Reproductive pattern	No true oestrous cycle	Seasonally polyoestrous: breeds from November to March	Seasonally polyoestrous: breeds from March to September	Polyoestrous	Polyoestrous	Polyoestrous	Polyoestrous	Polyoestrous
Length of oestrous cycle	Every 4 days	30–35 days	14 days	4–6 days	15–16 days	Every 4 days	4–5 days	4–5 days
Type of ovulation	Induced: occurs within 10 hours of mating	Spontaneous	Spontaneous	Spontaneous	Spontaneous	Spontaneous	Spontaneous	Spontaneous
Gestation period	28–32 days	111 days	28–32 days	24–26 days	63 days	15–18 days	19–21 days	20–22 days
Average litter size	2–7	2–3	2–6	3–6	2–6	3–7	6–12	6–12
Type of young at birth	Altricial	Precocial	Altricial	Altricial	Precocial	Altricial	Altricial	Altricial
Weaning age	4–6 weeks	6–8 weeks	6–7 weeks	3–4 weeks	3–4 weeks	3–4 weeks	18 days	3 weeks
Age of sexual maturity	5–8 months	8 months	12 months	10–12 weeks	6–10 weeks	6–10 weeks	3–4 weeks	5–6 weeks

15 REPTILES AND FISH

REPTILES

The class Reptilia includes about 6500 species, all of which breed on land. The class is divided into four orders of which only two are significant as far as exotic pets are concerned. The four orders are:

1. *Rhynchocephalia* – includes the tuatara; very rare and unlikely to be kept in captivity
2. *Crocodilia* – includes the crocodiles and alligators
3. *Chelonia* – includes tortoises, terrapins and turtles
4. *Squamata* – includes suborder *Sauria* (19 families of lizards), suborder *Serpentes* (11 families of snakes) and suborder *Amphisbaenia* (1 family, not kept in captivity).

These animals share many anatomical and physiological features so general reptilian anatomy and physiology will be discussed first, and any specific adaptations will be mentioned in the subsequent sections on lizards, snakes and the shelled reptiles (Chelonia).

General anatomy

Skeletal system

Reptiles are vertebrates and have an internal bony skeleton which, to some extent, shares the basic skeletal plan exhibited by members of the class Mammalia. However, there are distinctive modifications in the skeleton of the snakes, tortoises and turtles that will be discussed later.

Cardiovascular system

The *heart* has three chambers rather than four. There is a right and left atrium but only one ventricle. The ventricle is functionally, but not anatomically, divided into three sub-chambers and receives blood from both the right and left atria. Deoxygenated blood from the right atria is directed towards the pulmonary artery, but the oxygenated blood returning from the lungs to the ventricle may pass either to the aortic arches or to the pulmonary circulation again.

A significant feature of a reptile's peripheral circulation is the *renal portal system*, which transports blood from the hindlimbs and tail directly to the kidneys. This has clinical implications when injecting into the caudal half of the body, as some of the drug may be excreted in the urine before reaching the systemic circulation.

Respiratory system

Gaseous exchange occurs in the same way as it does in mammals but the most significant difference in the anatomy of the respiratory system of reptiles compared to that of mammals is that reptiles lack a *diaphragm*. As in the bird, the body cavity is not divided into two. Respiratory infections are common in reptiles but because they lack a diaphragm they lack an active, expulsive cough reflex and these infections can be severe or even fatal.

Digestive system

The more specific features of the digestive system of lizards, snakes and chelonians are covered separately. However, in general, the digestive system terminates in a common exit – the *cloaca*, consisting of three parts: the *coprodeum* collects the faeces, the *urodeum* collects urinary waste and the *proctodeum* is the final chamber that acts as a collecting area prior to the elimination of the waste.

Urinary system

The paired *kidneys* consist of nephrons without loops of Henle. This means that they are unable to produce concentrated urine. A thin walled *bladder* is present in lizards and Chelonia but is absent in snakes. The urine may change within the bladder so urinalysis in reptiles may not be an indication of kidney function, as it is in mammals.

Reproduction

Reptiles are *oviparous*, i.e. they lay eggs. The yolk of the egg provides the nourishment for the developing young, in contrast to mammals where the young are nourished directly by the mother via the placenta. Some reptiles are *ovoviviparous* or 'live-bearing' – they retain the developing young within the egg, which remains in the oviducts, and appear to give birth to live individuals. However, the nutrients are still obtained from the yolk of the egg inside which the young develop.

APPLIED ANATOMY

Dystocia or 'egg-binding' is commonly seen in reptiles. It can occur for a number of reasons, such as lack of a suitable nesting place, stress, calcium deficiency and infection.

The integument

The skin of reptiles is thick and keratinised and is protected by scales or horny plates. Reptiles grow by a process known as *ecdysis,* during which they shed or slough the old skin. Beneath this is a new layer which, to start with, is quite soft and easily damaged. Ecdysis varies with species and may be partial shedding, as seen in lizards, or entire, as seen in snakes.

Thermoregulation

Reptiles are *ectothermic,* i.e. they are unable to regulate their internal temperature and are dependent on the external environment to raise the body temperature and increase their metabolic rate. To do this they employ a number of behavioural patterns, e.g. basking in sunlight or spreading themselves as flat as possible in order to increase the surface area exposed to the sun. Each species has a preferred body temperature (PBT). This is the body temperature at which the reptile functions most efficiently. Below the PBT digestion is impaired and the immune system does not function so that reptiles kept at low temperatures are more likely to become ill.

TORTOISES, TERRAPINS AND TURTLES

Tortoises, turtles and terrapins are members of the order Chelonia (N.B. in the USA all shelled reptiles are referred to as turtles). They are characterised by a hard outer shell consisting of a domed upper part called the *carapace* and a flatter ventral part called the *plastron* (Fig. 15.1). The shell forms a bony 'box' that protects the soft internal parts of the body. The shell is covered with horny plates or *scutes,* which are named according to the most adjacent part of the body. The scutes grow from the outside so that an annual ring develops along the periphery of each one making the overall shell larger. In some species these 'growth rings' can be used to estimate age.

Anatomical features

Skeleton

Chelonians are vertebrates and their skeleton resembles that of other vertebrates. However, the pectoral and pelvic girdles are within the rib cage and are orientated vertically to buttress the shell (Fig. 15.1). The ten vertebrae form part of the under surface of the carapace.

Cardiovascular system

Chelonians possess the normal reptilian three-chambered heart and renal portal system. The outer shell of chelonians makes auscultation of the heart difficult, but may be aided by putting a damp towel around the shell.

Respiratory system

The rigid outer shell of chelonians prevents the body wall from expanding during breathing. Respiration is accomplished with the aid of limb and head movements, which move in and out and alter the internal pressure in the body cavity. Chelonians breathe through their external nares or nostrils, so mouth breathing may indicate a respiratory problem. The glottis lies at the base of the tongue, and the trachea is short which allows the tortoise to breathe when the neck is withdrawn. The lungs are positioned dorsally, below the carapace, and aid buoyancy in aquatic species (Fig. 15.1).

Digestive system

Chelonians do not have teeth and depend on their horny beak to cut off pieces of food. They have large, fleshy tongues that cannot protrude from the mouth. The oesophagus runs down the left side of the neck and joins the stomach, which lies transversely across the body (Fig. 15.2). The small intestine is relatively short (compared to mammals), and the colon ends in the *cloaca,* which is the common chamber into which the urogenital and digestive systems empty.

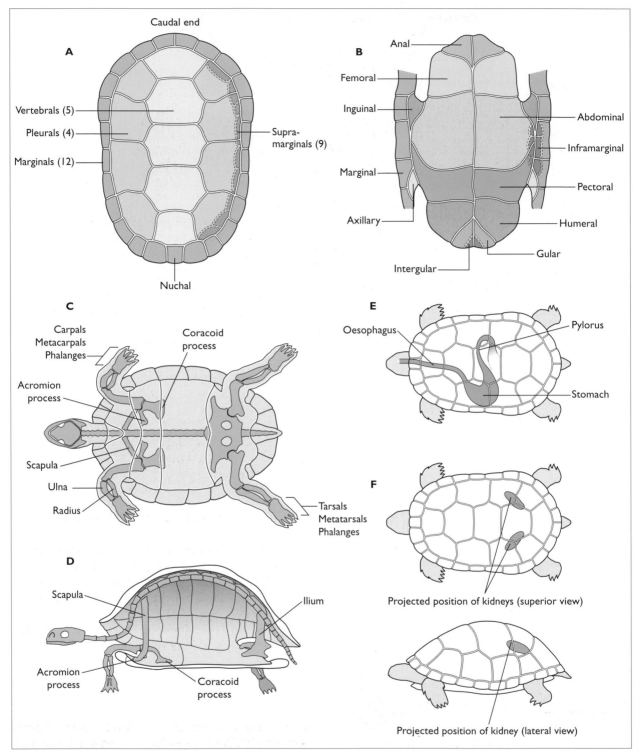

Fig. 15.1 Anatomy of the tortoise (*Testudo spp.*). **A** Carapace. **B** Plastron. **C** Ventral view of skeleton. **D** Left side view of skeleton. **E** First part of intestinal tract. **F** Position of the kidneys.

Urogenital system

In chelonians the ureters conduct relatively uncon-centrated urine from the kidneys into a thin-walled urinary bladder (Fig. 15.2). Male chelonians possess a single, large penis that protrudes from the floor of the cloaca.

Sexual differentiation

Most species of Chelonia are sexually dimorphic: there are visible differences in external features such as colouration, tail length, shell size and shape. Features include:

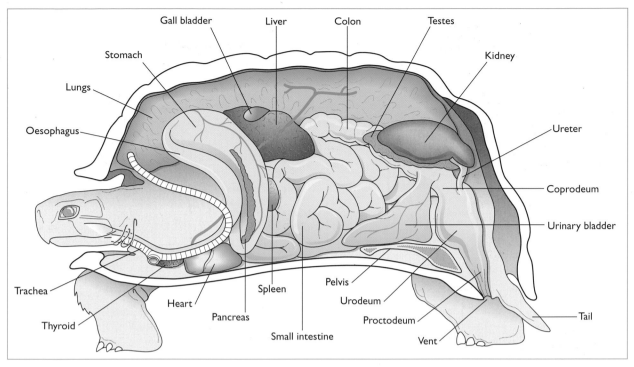

Fig. 15.2 Internal anatomy of the tortoise.

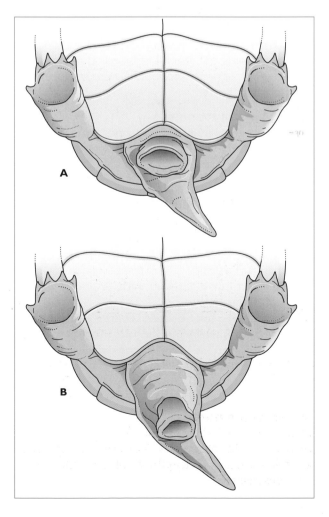

Fig. 15.3 Determining the sex of chelonians. **A** Female. **B** Male. The tail of the male is longer, the plastron is concave and the cloacal opening is further down on the tail.

1. Male tortoises have longer tails than females (Fig. 15.3).
2. The plastron of the male is concave to enable him to mount the domed carapace of the female.
3. The caudal scute of the female may be curved upwards to allow her to elevate her tail during mating.
4. The male terrapin has long front claws with which he 'tickles' the chin of the female.

LIZARDS

Lizards belong to the suborder *Sauria*, which includes about 3750 different species classified into 19 families.

Anatomical features

Skeleton

The skeleton of the lizard follows the basic vertebrate plan, but there is no sternum (Fig. 15.4). Most lizards have four legs and most species take their weight on all their legs, however some species, e.g. the basilisk, can run on two legs. The anatomy of the limbs indicates the mode of locomotion.

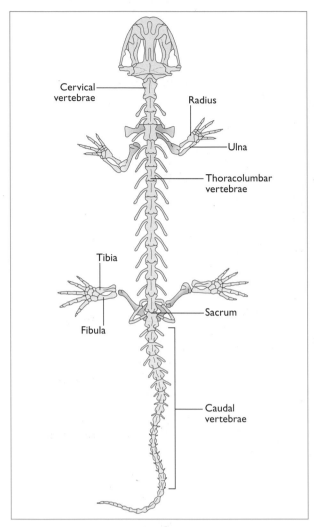

Fig. 15.4 Skeleton of a lizard.

APPLIED ANATOMY

Many species of lizard show *autotomy*. This is the ability to shed their tail as a defence against predators. Once shed, the tail keeps squirming and distracts the predator while the lizard runs away! A replacement tail may grow but it is often a different colour and may be shrunken; internally the replacement vertebrae are cartilaginous rather than bony. If a lizard is stressed or if the tail is damaged it may fall off – this must be considered when handling or injecting into the tail muscle. As a result of autotomy the tail muscles go into spasm and prevent excessive blood loss.

Integument

Lizards have thick scaly skin and grow by shedding the skin *(ecdysis)*. In lizards the skin comes off in pieces and some species will eat the sloughed pieces. The family *Skinkidae* – the skinks – shed their skin in one piece; they are covered in scales that fit tightly together producing a smooth streamlined outline. Some species of lizard, e.g. chameleons, are able to change the colour of their skin. This is due to the presence of *chromatophores* in the skin and helps to camouflage the lizard. Members of the family *Gekkonidae* – the geckos – are characterised by having layers of overlapping scales or lamellae on the underside of their feet. This enables them to grip on to apparently smooth surfaces such as glass.

Special senses

The *ear* is responsible for both hearing and balance. The tympanic membrane is easily visible in a shallow depression on the side of the head and is covered by a thin layer of skin that is shed periodically with the rest of the skin. The *eye* is protected by an eyelid in most species of lizard and in some species the lower lid is transparent to allow vision even when the lids are closed.

Cardiovascular system

Lizards possess the typical reptilian *three-chambered heart* and the *renal portal system* as previously described. They have a large ventral abdominal vein and care must be taken when making a midline incision. The ventral tail vein may be used for venepuncture, but should not be used in species that are able to shed the tail. In larger species the cephalic vein on the forelimb may be used.

Respiratory system

The diaphragm is absent and breathing is accomplished by expansion and contraction of the ribs.

Digestive system

Most lizards possess *teeth* that are attached to the sides of the mandible and not in sockets as seen in mammals. These teeth are regularly shed and then replaced. In some families of lizard, e.g. chameleons, the teeth are attached to the biting edges of the jaw and these are not shed. The *tongue* is used to 'taste' the environment in conjunction with *Jacobsen's organ* in the roof of the mouth.

The digestive tract of lizards varies depending on the type of diet, which may be insectivorous, carnivorous, herbivorous or omnivorous depending on the species (Fig. 15.5). The *stomach* is simple and elongated, and a *caecum* is present in herbivorous species. The digestive tract terminates in the typical reptilian *cloaca*.

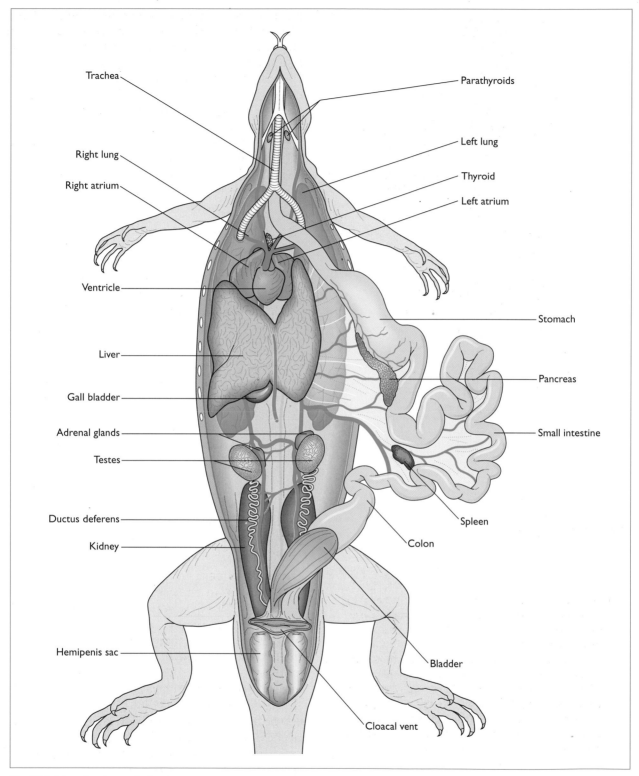

Fig. 15.5 Internal anatomy of a lizard.

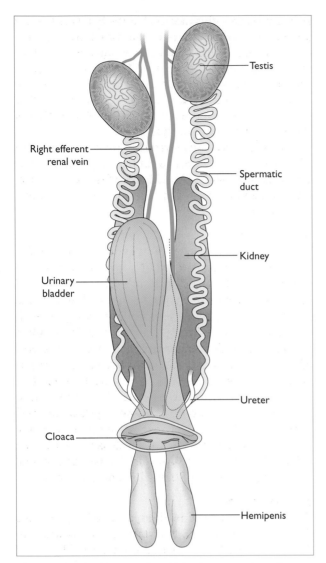

Fig. 15.6 Urogenital system of a male lizard.

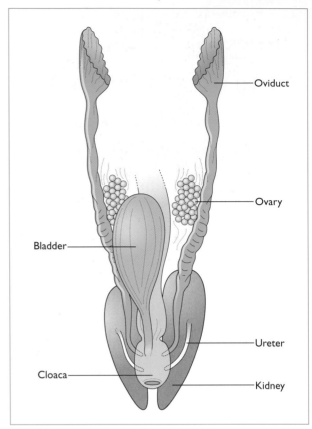

Fig. 15.7 Urogenital system of a female lizard.

Some species of lizard consist entirely of females and reproduction is by means of *parthenogenesis* in which the young develop from an unfertilised egg – they are all female.

Urogenital system

Most species of lizard possess a urinary bladder (Fig. 15.5). *Male* lizards possess paired copulatory organs, called *hemipenes* (Fig. 15.6). Each hemipenis is a hollow structure with a closed end, which lies invaginated in the base of the tail, posterior to the cloaca. The hemipenes are stored in an inverted position in the base of the tail. Only one hemipenis is used during copulation and is erected by filling with blood. It is then inserted into the cloaca of the female. The shape of the hemipenes varies with the species. *Female* lizards lay eggs. They have a pair of ovaries and oviducts but there is no uterus. The eggs pass out of the body via the cloaca (Fig. 15.7).

Sexual differentiation

The method of determining the sex of a lizard is dependent on the species.

1. *Sexual dimorphism* – many species show differences in shape and colour between the two sexes. Males may also show display patterns such as flashing colours or the use of erectable crests to attract the female.
2. *Base of the tail* – males may have a more swollen base to their tail, inside which is lie hemipenes.
3. *Presence of femoral or preanal pores* (Fig. 15.8) – different species show various patterns of pores on the inner surface of the inguinal region.

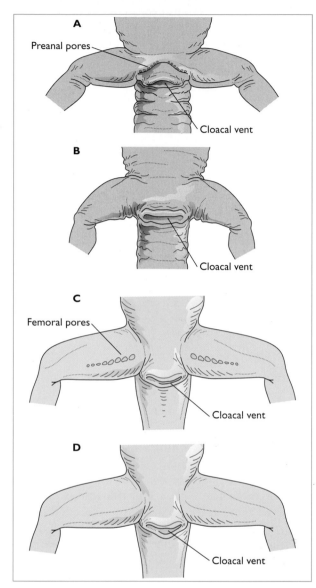

Fig. 15.8 Sexual differentiation in lizards. **A**, **B** Geckos: males have anal or preanal pores in the inguinal region. **C**, **D** Agamas: males have femoral pores.

SNAKES

Snakes belong to the suborder *Serpentes* which includes around 2400 species divided between 11 different families.

Anatomical features

Skeleton

Snakes are legless and have an elongated body (Fig. 15.9). They have a complex skull, which is described as being *kinetic* – this means that the bones of the jaw are loosely connected and the two halves of the mandible are joined by an elastic ligament to allow wide separation (Fig. 15.10). These features enable the snake to ingest large items of prey. Snakes do not have thoracic limbs but a few possess vestigial pelvic limbs, seen as external spurs in the pelvic region of species such as boas and pythons.

The snake has many *vertebrae* – numbers vary from 150 to over 400 – all with a similar shape. Each vertebra gives off a pair of ribs which are fused to the vertebra but are not joined in the ventral midline, i.e. there is no sternum.

Integument

The epidermal scales of the integument show differences according to the region of the body. In the dorsal and lateral parts of the body the scales are small and on the ventral surface they are larger and thicker. The tough, smooth skin of the snake does not grow with the snake but is shed periodically, usually in one piece to reveal a new skin underneath *(ecdysis)*. At the time of shedding the snake skin may have a dull appearance due to the lifting of the old outer layer of skin. Snakes do not have moveable eyelids, as are seen in mammals, but the upper and lower eyelids are fused together to form a transparent *spectacle* over the cornea. During ecdysis the spectacle is also shed. Just before shedding the snake may be withdrawn and anorexic and handling should be kept to a minimum.

Special senses

The eyes are protected by the spectacle lying over the surface of the cornea. Tear-like secretions are produced between the cornea and spectacle. The ear of the snake has no tympanic membrane and no middle ear cavity. Some species of snake, e.g. members of the family *Boidae* – the boas – have heat sensitive pits on the upper jaw which are used to detect their prey. These are so sensitive that they can pick up heat changes of 0.001°C.

Cardiovascular system

Snakes possess the typical reptilian *heart,* and have both *renal* and *hepatic portal* circulations. The heart is generally located at about one third of the length of the body.

Respiratory system

In most snakes the *left lung* is greatly reduced in size or even absent (Fig 15.11). Only the anterior part of the lung is functional for gaseous exchange. The posterior part is avascular and functions as an air sac that may act as a reserve during periods of apnoea.

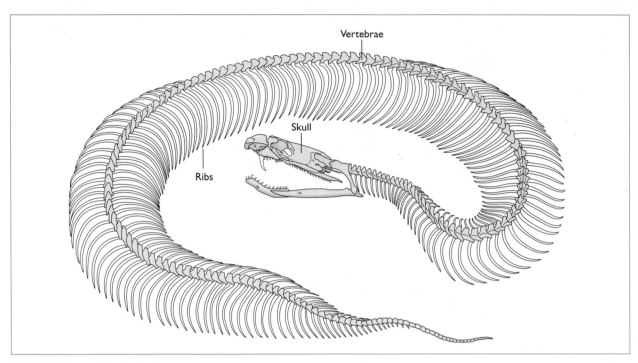

Fig. 15.9 Skeleton of a typical snake.

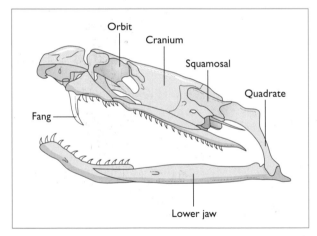

Fig. 15.10 The bones of a snake skull.

Digestive system

Snakes are totally carnivorous and possess six rows of undifferentiated *teeth* which are replaced continuously (Fig. 15.10). Some species may have modified *fangs* and some are able to produce *venom* from special glands that lie above the oral cavity. The venom is delivered to the prey by the fangs. The *tongue* is thin, forked and mobile and is able to protrude some distance out of the mouth. It is used for olfaction – the snake 'tastes' the environment and the tongue is then brought into contact with *Jacobsen's organ* in the roof of the mouth, and information is conveyed by a branch of the olfactory nerve to the brain. As the body of the snake is long and thin the organs are arranged along its length rather than across the body (Fig. 15.11). The *stomach* is elongated but the *intestines* are relatively short, reflecting the carnivorous diet.

Urogenital system

There is no urinary bladder in snakes and the ureters empty into the *urodeum* section of the *cloaca*. Male snakes possess invaginated *hemipenes* that lie in the base of the tail just caudal to the vent. The hemipenis evaginates into the cloaca of the female to transmit sperm during copulation. Females of very slender species of snake have only one oviduct and ovary.

Sexual differentiation

The method used to determine the sex of a snake depends on its species.

1. *Sexual dimorphism* – in some species it is possible to differentiate between the sexes by looking at the colour and the markings.
2. *Tail length* – the tail is measured from the vent (the exit of the cloaca) to the tip of the tail. The male

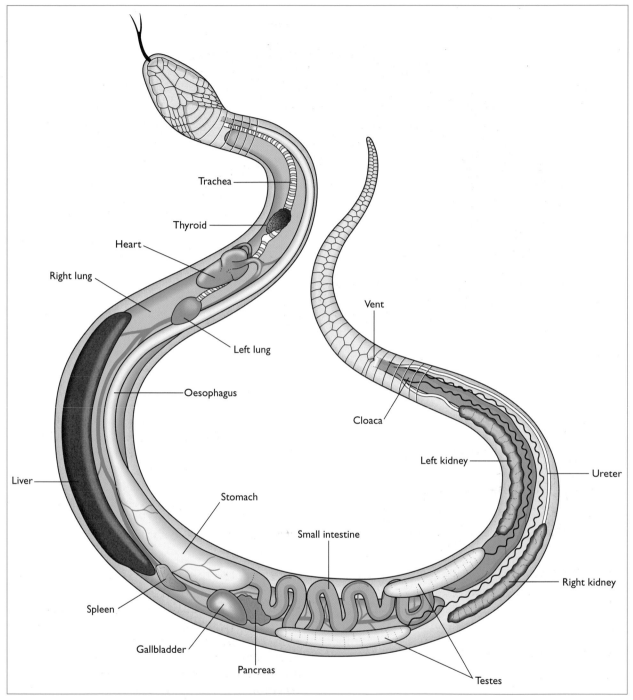

Fig. 15.11 Internal anatomy of a snake.

usually has a longer tail than the female and the area around the vent may be noticeably swollen. This area houses the hemipenes.

3. *Size* – in some species the female is larger than the male.

4. *Use of a probe* – this requires experience and great care. A well lubricated blunt-ended rod is carefully introduced into the cloaca pointing towards the tail. In the male, the probe will travel a longer distance down the cloaca than it does in the female.

FISH

Fish are *ectothermic* vertebrates that live and breathe in water and move with the aid of fins. There are over 30 000 species of fish, which makes them the most numerous of vertebrates. They range in size from the tiny Philippine Island goby, which measures less than 1 cm, to the whale shark, which measures up to 16 m. There are two groups of jawed fish: the *cartilaginous fish* (sharks and rays) and the *bony fish*, which includes all the ornamental fish likely to be kept in captivity. Within the bony fish are the group known as the *teleosts*, which comprises 20 000 species divided into the *lower Teleosts*, e.g. carp, salmon and catfish, and the *higher teleosts*, e.g. perch, sticklebacks and mackerel. They are found in a wide range of habitats all over the world. Many groups of fish kept in captivity have been selectively bred, e.g. goldfish, which has led to the development of an enormous range of fins, eyes, colour, tails and size. However, all teleosts have a similar general structure.

General anatomy

Musculoskeletal system

The *fusiform* shape of a fish makes it streamlined for swimming. Locomotion is facilitated by muscle blocks or *myomeres* arranged on either side of the axial skeleton (Fig. 15.12). This enables the body to bend laterally and generate the propulsive force to move forward. The *cranium* is rigid and articulates with the bones of the jaws and opercula apparatus. The number of *vertebrae* varies; ribs in the thoracic region articulate with the vertebrae and support the lateral walls of the body cavity.

Fish possess *fins*, which are responsible for the fish's ability to manoeuvre and remain stable in the water. The fins consist of tissue stretched between rays which may be stiff and unjointed or soft with many articulations (Fig. 15.13). The fins are attached to small muscles which fold or extend the fins to produce rapid precise movements. The shape of the *caudal fin* or *tail* provides an indication of the swimming habits of the fish, e.g. a forked tail enables the fish to swim at continuous high speeds, while a truncated tail is seen in slow moving species and allows them to make fast dashes.

Buoyancy in the water is achieved by a gas-filled *swim bladder* in the body of the fish, below the vertebral column (Fig. 15.14). The specific gravity of the teleosts is greater than that of the surrounding water so there is a tendency to sink if they remain stationary. By altering the volume of air in the swim bladder the fish can rise and remain in one place – they achieve neutral buoyancy despite pressure changes in the water. The swim bladder has evolved from the primitive lung of the lower teleosts and is a thin-walled diverticulum of the foregut. The structure varies depending on the species:

- *Lower teleosts* – the swim bladder is linked via a pneumatic duct to the foregut and is described as being *physostomous*. This type occurs mainly in shallow freshwater species. The swim bladder is

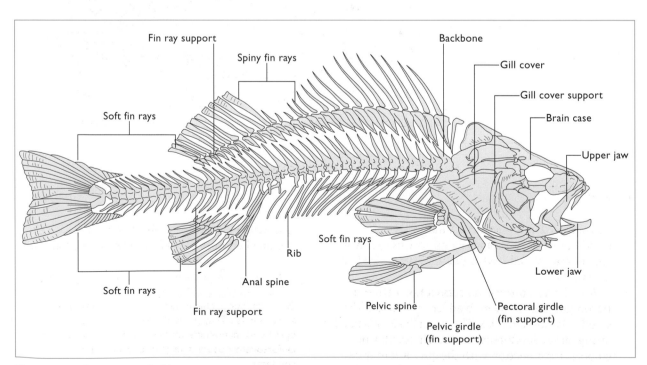

Fig. 15.12 Skeletal structure of a fish.

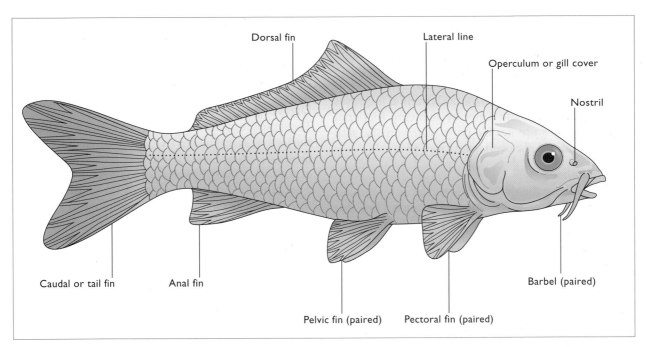

Fig. 15.13 External anatomy of a fish.

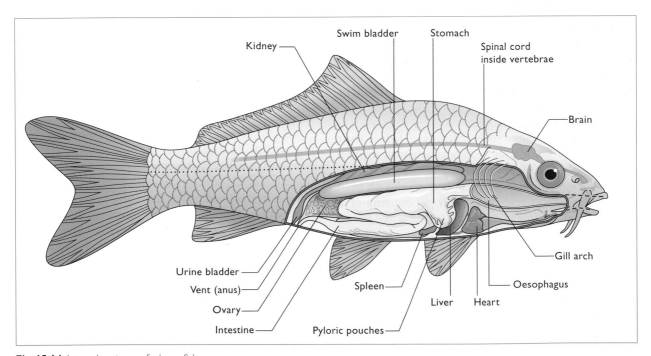

Fig. 15.14 Internal anatomy of a bony fish.

refilled by rising to the surface and taking a mouthful of air. In bottom-living species the swim bladder may be reduced, enabling them to feed on the river bed.

■ *Higher teleosts* – there is no connection between the foregut and the swim bladder and the bladder is said to be *physoclistous*. The swim bladder is filled during larval development, when there may be a temporary connection with the gut, or it may be filled by a gas gland within the cells of the sac. The

gas, which consists mainly of carbon dioxide, is retained in the sac for life by its impermeable walls.

APPLIED ANATOMY

Swim bladder problems are relatively common in aquarium fish. They present as an inability to float upright, to manoeuvre or to swim below the surface. Unfortunately there is very little treatment for the condition.

REFERENCES AND RECOMMENDED READING

REFERENCES

Adams, D.R. (1986) *Canine Anatomy*. Iowa: Iowa State University Press.

Aspinall, V. (2001) *Anatomy and Physiology for Veterinary Nurses* (Vetlogic Series of CD ROMS). Stroud: Keyskills Co. Ltd.

Beaver, B.V. (1992) *Feline Behaviour*. Philadelphia: W.B. Saunders.

Beynon, P. (ed) (1996) *Manual of Psittacine Birds*. Gloucester: BSAVA.

Beynon, P. & Cooper, J.E. (eds) (1992) *Manual of Exotic Pets*. Gloucester: BSAVA.

Beynon, P., Lawton, M.P.C. & Cooper, J.E. (1992) *Manual of Reptiles*. Gloucester: BSAVA.

Bowden, C. & Masters, J. (eds) (2001) *Pre-Veterinary Nursing Textbook*. Oxford: Butterworth Heinemann.

Boyd, J.S. (2001) *Colour Atlas of Clinical Anatomy of the Dog and Cat*, 2nd edn. London: Mosby.

Butcher, R.L. (ed) *Manual of Ornamental Fish*. Gloucester: BSAVA.

Colville, T. & Bassett, J.M. (2002) *Clinical Anatomy and Physiology for Veterinary Technicians*. St Louis: Mosby.

Cooper, J.E. (2002) *Birds of Prey – Health and Disease*. Oxford: Blackwell Scientific Publications.

Dyce, K.M., Sack, W.O. & Wensing, C.J.G. (1996) *Textbook of Veterinary Anatomy*, 2nd edn. Philadelphia: W.B. Saunders.

Evans, H.E. (1993) *Miller's Anatomy of the Dog*, 3rd edn. Philadelphia: W.B. Saunders.

Evans, J.M. & White, K. (1988) *The Book of the Bitch*. Guildford: Henston.

Flecknell, P. (ed) (2000) *Manual of Rabbit Medicine and Surgery*. Gloucester: BSAVA.

Frandson, R.D. & Spurgeon, T.L. (1992) *Anatomy and Physiology of Farm Animals*. Philadelphia: Lea and Febiger.

Freeman, W.H. & Bracegirdle, B. (1966) *Atlas of Histology*. London: Heinemann.

Fullick, A. (2000) *Biology*. Oxford: Heinemann.

Harvey Pough, F., Heiser, J.B. & McFarland, W.N. (1993) *Vertebrate Life*, 3rd edn. Basingstoke: Macmillan.

Hillyer, E.V. & Quesenberry, K.E. (1997) *Ferrets, Rabbits and Rodents – Clinical Medicine and Surgery*. Philadelphia: WB Saunders.

King, A.S. & McClelland, J. (1984) *Birds – Their Structure and Function*. London: Balliere Tindall.

Laber-Laird, K., Swindle, M.M. & FLecknell, P. (eds) (1996) *Handbook of Rodent and Rabbit Medicine*. Oxford: Pergamon.

Lane, D.R. (1991) *Jones' Animal Nursing*, 5th edn. Oxford: Pergamon.

Lane, D.R. & Cooper, B. (eds) (1999) *Veterinary Nursing*, 2nd edn. Oxford: Butterworth Heinemann.

Mader, D.R. (1996) *Reptile Medicine and Surgery*. Philadelphia: W.B. Saunders.

McArthur, S. (1996) *Veterinary Management of Tortoises and Turtles*. Oxford: Blackwell Science.

Meredith, A. & Redrobe, S. (eds) (2002) *Manual of Exotic Pets*, 4th edn. Gloucester: BSAVA.

Michell, A.R. & Watkins, P.E. (1989) *An Introduction to Anatomy and Physiology*. Gloucester: BSAVA.

Okerman, L. (1994) *Diseases of Domestic Rabbits*. Oxford: Blackwell Science.

Phillips, W.D. & Chilton, T.J. (1989) *A-Level Biology*. Oxford: Oxford University Press.

Pickering, W.R. (1996) *Advanced Human Biology*. Oxford: Oxford University Press.

Roberts, M.B.V. (1986) *Biology – A Functional Approach*. 4th edn. Walton-on-Thames: Nelson.

Roberts, R.J. (ed) (2001) *Fish Pathology*, 3rd edn. Philadelphia: W.B. Saunders.

Ruckebusch, Y., Phaneuf, L-P. & Dunlop, R. (1991) *Physiology of Small and Large Animals*. Philadelphia: B.C. Decker.

Shively, M.J. & Beaver, B.G. (1985) *Dissection of the Dog and Cat*. Iowa: Iowa State University Press.

Smith, B.J. (1999) *Canine Anatomy*. Philadelphia: Lippincott, Williams and Wilkins.

Sturkie, P.D. (ed) (1976) *Avian Physiology*. New York: Springer Verlag.

Turner, T. (1994) *Veterinary Notes for Dog Owners*. London: Popular Dogs.

Warren Dean, M. (1995) *Small Animal Care and Management*. New York: Delmar Publishers.

RECOMMENDED READING

Aspinall, V. (2001) *Anatomy and Physiology for Veterinary Nurses* (Vetlogic Series of CD ROMS). Stroud: Keyskills Co. Ltd.

Boyd, J.S. (2001) *Colour Atlas of Clinical Anatomy of the Dog and Cat,* 2nd edn. London: Mosby.

Colville, T. & Bassett, J.M. (2002) *Clinical Anatomy and Physiology for Veterinary Technicians.* St Louis: Mosby.

Lane, D.R. & Cooper, B. (eds) (2003) *Veterinary Nursing,* 3rd edn. Oxford: Butterworth Heinemann.

Smith, B.J. (1999) *Canine Anatomy.* Philadelphia: Lippincott, Williams and Wilkins.

Tartaglia, L. & Waugh, A. (2002) *Veterinary Physiology and Applied Anatomy.* Oxford: Butterworth Heinemann.

INTRODUCTION TO ANATOMICAL TERMINOLOGY

Many of the words used in anatomy and physiology will be unfamiliar to you and may often appear rather daunting. However, if you become aware of the concept of breaking down a word into its component parts then the word can be 'dissected' to discover its meaning. This technique is useful when trying to understand the veterinary 'jargon' used by vets as well as within the broader context of anatomy and physiology.

A *prefix* is found at the beginning of a word, e.g. *peri* in pericardium. The prefix itself has a general meaning, e.g. *peri* means 'around', but when combined with another word it gives a specific meaning: pericardium meaning literally 'around the heart'. Prefixes are given in Table A.1.

A *suffix* is found at the end of a word, e.g. *cyte* in osteocyte. Suffixes also have a general meaning, e.g. *cyte* means cell, but when added to a word it becomes specific: osteocyte meaning bone cell. Suffixes are given in Table A.2.

The *root* of a word is the essence of its meaning, e.g. peri*cardium*. The root often refers to the organ, structure or disease in question; the root *cardium* relates to the heart. It can be considered as the 'word element', which is often derived from a Latin or Greek word. Roots are given in Table A.3.

Other words simply have a meaning that can be used within a word, e.g. *genesis* means 'creation or origination'. Thus, *carcinogenic* means that something 'creates' cancer; similarly, *pathogenic* means 'causing disease'.

Table A.1 Common prefixes.

Prefix	Meaning	Examples
A-	Without; not	*Avascular* – without a blood supply
Anti-	Working against; counteracting	*Antibody* – neutralises antigens; *antiseptic* – inhibits growth of bacteria; *antihistamine* – inhibits the effects of histamine
Ante- (also **Pre-**)	Before	*Anterior* – structures at the front of the body; *antenatal* – before parturition; *prepubic* – in front of the pubis
Brady-	Slow	*Bradycardia* – slow heart rate; *bradypnoea* – slower than normal breathing
Cyto-	A cell	*Cytotoxic* – something that has a damaging effect on cells (e.g. cytotoxic drugs)
Dys-	Difficult; impaired	*Dyspnoea* – difficulty in breathing; *dysplasia* – an abnormality of development
Endo-	Within	*Endometrium* – the inner lining of the uterus; *endothelium* – the layer of epithelial cells that lines the inside of the heart and blood vessels
Epi-	Upon; outside of	*Epidermis* – the outermost layer of the skin; *epiglottis* – cartilaginous structure that guards the entrance to the larynx
Erythr(o)-	Red	*Erythrocyte* – red blood cell; *erythema* – redness of the skin
Hyper-	Excessive; increased	*Hypertensive* – high blood pressure; *hypertrophy* – increase in the size of a tissue or organ
Hypo-	Decreased; deficient; beneath	*Hypothermia* – low body temperature; *hypodermis* – the subcutis that lies beneath the skin
Peri-	Around; in the region of	*Periosteum* – the connective tissue that surrounds a bone; *perianal* – around the anus
Poly-	Many; much	*Polyoestrous* – having more than one oestrous cycle a year; *polyarthritis* – inflammation of several joints; *polypeptide* – a compound containing three or more linked amino acids
Post-	After; behind	*Postmortem* – after death; *postoperative* – after a surgical operation; *posterior* – towards the rear
Pyo-	Pus	*Pyometra* – presence of pus in the uterus; *pyoderma* – bacterial infection of the skin
Tachy-	Rapid	*Tachycardia* – elevated heart rate

Table A.2 Common suffixes.

Suffix	Meaning	Examples
-aemia	Relates to the blood	*Ischaemia* – reduced or deficient blood supply; *viraemia* – the presence of virus particles in the bloodstream
-cyte [Cyt(o) is the prefix used]	A cell	*Erythrocyte* – red blood cell; *chondrocyte* – cartilage cell; *hepatocyte* – liver cell
-ectomy	Surgical removal of	*Thyroidectomy* – removal of the thyroid gland
-genic	Giving rise to; causing	*Pathogenic* – causing disease; *carcinogenic* – causing neoplasia or cancer
-ia/-iasis	Condition or state	*Hypoplasia* – incomplete development of an organ or tissue; *distichiasis* – presence of a double row of eyelashes
-itis	Inflammation	*Arthritis* – inflammation of a joint; *hepatitis* – inflammation of the liver; *conjunctivitis* – inflammation of the conjunctiva of the eye
-oma	Tumour, neoplasm	*Sarcoma* – malignant tumour; *lipoma* – benign tumour of adipose tissue
-osis	Disease order or state	*Osteochondrosis* – a developmental disease of articular cartilage
-ostomy	Surgical opening	*Tracheostomy* – opening into the trachea; *colostomy* – opening into the colon

Table A.3 Common roots of words.

Root word	Meaning	Examples
Arthr(o)	Joint; articulation	*Arthrodesis* – surgical fusion of a joint; *arthritis* – inflammation of a joint
Cardi(o)	Heart	*Cardiology* – the study of the heart and its function; *myocardium* – muscle layer of the heart
Chondro	Cartilage	*Chondrocyte* – cartilage cell; *perichondrium* – membrane that covers cartilage
Cyst(o)	Bladder	*Cystotomy* – incision into the bladder; *cystitis* – inflammation of the urinary bladder
Dermat(o)	Skin	*Dermatitis* – inflammation of the skin
Gloss(o) (also **lingual**)	Tongue	*Hypoglossal* – situated below the tongue (also *sublingual*)
Haemat(o) /**Haem**(o)	Blood	*Haematemesis* – vomiting blood; *haemorrhage* – the escape of blood from a ruptured vessel
Hepat(o)	Liver	*Hepatocyte* – liver cell; *hepatic artery* – artery that supplies blood to the liver
Hist(io/o)	Tissue	*Histology* – the study of tissues
Mamm(o) (also **masto**)	Breast; mammary gland	*Mammogram* – radiograph of a mammary gland; *mastectomy* – surgical removal of mammary gland
Metra-/metro	Uterus	*Endometrium* – lining of the uterus; *metritis* – inflammation of the uterus
Myo-	Muscle	*Myositis* – inflammation of a voluntary muscle
Neur(o)	Nerve	*Neuralgia* – pain in a nerve; *neuron* – nerve cell
Ophthalm(o)	Eye	*Ophthalmoscope* – instrument used to examine the interior of the eye
Orchi	Testis (testicle)	*Orchitis* – inflammation of a testis; *cryptorchid* – having an undescended testicle
Oste(o)	Bone	*Osteomyelitis* – inflammation of bone
Pneum(o)	Air or gas; lung	*Pneumonia* – inflammation of the lung tissue; *pneumothorax* – the presence of free air in the thorax
-pnoea	Respiration; breathing	*Apnoea* – temporary cessation in breathing
Ren-	Kidney	*Renal artery* – the artery that supplies the kidney with blood
Rhin(o)	Nose	*Rhinitis* – inflammation of the mucous membrane of the nose
Trich(o)	Hair	*Trichosis* – any disease of, or abnormal growth of hair
Vas(o)	Vessel; duct	*Vascular* – pertaining to blood vessels; *vasoconstriction* – decrease in the diameter of a blood vessel; *vasectomy* – excision of the vas deferens (deferent duct)

MULTIPLE CHOICE QUESTIONS

These multiple choice questions are based on the facts in the book, so why not test your understanding of what you have read? There is one correct answer to each question. The answers can be found on page 224.

Section 1–The Dog and Cat

1. Principles of Cell Biology

1.1 The cell membrane is mainly composed of:
a. a single layer of protein molecules
b. a protein bilayer
c. a phospholipid bilayer
d. a polysaccharide bilayer

1.2 Which of the following is *not* found in the nucleus of the cell?
a. centrioles
b. chromosomes
c. DNA
d. nucleoli

1.3 Which organelle is the site for ATP production?
a. nucleoli
b. mitochondria
c. golgi complex
d. ribosomes

1.4 What is the function of the rough endoplasmic reticulum in the mammalian cell?
a. storage of lysosomal enzymes
b. synthesis and transport of proteins
c. synthesis of glucose
d. production of ATP

1.5 During which stage of mitosis do the chromosomes line up in the middle of the cell?
a. prophase
b. anaphase
c. metaphase
d. telophase

1.6 When does 'crossing-over' take place during meiosis?
a. metaphase
b. prophase
c. anaphase
d. telophase

1.7 Fluid that has a lower osmotic pressure than that of plasma is said to be:
a. hypotonic
b. isotonic
c. hypertonic
d. isometric

1.8 Which of the following cations is in a relatively higher concentration in the intracellular fluid than in the extracellular fluid?
a. potassium
b. iodine
c. sodium
d. chloride

1.9 Which of the following is *not* an example of a structural protein?
a. collagen
b. enzymes
c. elastin
d. keratin

1.10 Which of the following statements is the least accurate?
a. an acidic solution has a pH of below 7
b. the pH scale is a measure of a solution's hydrogen ion content
c. an alkaline substance releases hydrogen ions when dissolved in a solution
d. the pH of body fluids is 7.35

2. The Tissues and Body Cavities

2.1   Which of the following is *not* a connective tissue?
   a. bone
   b. cartilage
   c. muscle
   d. blood

2.2   Which type of tissue covers the external and internal surfaces of the body?
   a. connective
   b. skin
   c. areolar
   d. epithelial

2.3   Where would you find simple cuboidal epithelium?
   a. lining the bladder
   b. lining the upper respiratory tract
   c. lining the renal nephron
   d. in the epidermis

2.4   What type of epithelium lines the ureters?
   a. simple squamous
   b. ciliated columnar
   c. transitional
   d. stratified squamous

2.5   Which of the following is an example of a simple coiled gland?
   a. salivary
   b. sweat
   c. duodenal
   d. sebaceous

2.6   Which type of cartilage is found in the epiglottis?
   a. hyaline
   b. fibrous
   c. elastic
   d. globular

2.7   Which type of bone tissue is found in the cortices of all types of bone?
   a. spongy
   b. cancellous
   c. hyaline
   d. compact

2.8   The contractile protein that makes up the thin filaments of a muscle fibre is:
   a. actin
   b. elastin
   c. collagen
   d. myosin

2.9   What is the name given to the serous endothelium that lines the inside of the thoracic cavity?
   a. parietal peritoneum
   b. parietal pleura
   c. visceral peritoneum
   d. mediastinum

2.10 What is found within the peritoneal cavity?
   a. pleural fluid
   b. the pericardium
   c. peritoneal fluid
   d. the mediastinum

3. The Skeletal System

3.1   Which of the following is a splanchnic bone?
a. tuber calcis
b. patella
c. os penis
d. calcaneus

3.2   Where do the primary centres of ossification appear in a long bone?
a. the diaphysis
b. the ends
c. the epiphyses
d. the epiphyseal plate

3.3   Which bone of the skull lies at the base of the orbit and is the region through which the tears drain into the nose?
a. sphenoid
b. ethmoid
c. occipital
d. lacrimal

3.4   Which of the following joints is an example of an amphiarthrosis?
a. the temporomandibular
b. sutures of the skull
c. between the bodies of the vertebrae
d. between the skull and the atlas

3.5   Which part of the mandible articulates with the temporal region of the skull?
a. masseteric fossa
b. condylar process
c. coronoid process
d. occipital condyle

3.6   Which part of a thoracic vertebra articulates with the tubercle of a rib?
a. the spinous process
b. the costal fovea
c. the transverse fovea
d. neural arch

3.7   How many sternebrae is the sternum comprised of?
a. 7
b. 13
c. 3
d. 8

3.8   The olecranon fossa receives which part of the ulna during extension of the elbow?
a. olecranon
b. anconeal process
c. coronoid process
d. styloid process

3.9   On which bone would you find the medial malleolus?
a. tibia
b. fibula
c. femur
d. radius

3.10 How many short bones are found in the tarsus?
a. 5
b. 7
c. 3
d. 2

4. The Muscular System

4.1   What is the unit of contraction in a muscle called?
   a. motor unit
   b. sarcomere
   c. origin
   d. insertion

4.2   Which of the following muscles protracts the forelimb and bends the neck laterally?
   a. brachialis
   b. biceps brachii
   c. brachiocephalicus
   d. biceps femoris

4.3   Which muscle inserts on the coronoid process of the mandible?
   a. temporalis
   b. masseter
   c. digastricus
   d. pterygoid

4.4   Where do the extra-ocular muscles insert?
   a. linea alba
   b. optic foramen
   c. the orbit
   d. the sclera

4.5   Through which of the openings in the diaphragm does the thoracic duct pass?
   a. oesophageal hiatus
   b. aortic hiatus
   c. inguinal ring
   d. caval foramen

4.6   Which of the following muscles does *not* insert on the linea alba?
   a. external abdominal oblique
   b. transversus abdominis
   c. rectus abdominus
   d. internal abdominal oblique

4.7   Which muscle inserts on the spine of the scapula?
   a. trapezius
   b. infraspinatus
   c. pectorals
   d. latissimus dorsi

4.8   The patella is found in the tendon of insertion of which muscle?
   a. biceps femoris
   b. gastrocnemius
   c. semitendinosis
   d. quadriceps femoris

4.9   Which muscle flexes the hock?
   a. gastrocnemius
   b. biceps femoris
   c. anterior tibialis
   d. pectineus

4.10 Which of the following muscles is *not* a component of the Achilles tendon?
   a. semimembranosus
   b. biceps femoris
   c. semitendinosus
   d. superficial digital flexor

5. The Nervous System and Special Senses

5.1   Which of the following structures is *not* part of the peripheral nervous system?
a. cranial nerve V
b. spinal nerves supplying the intercostal muscles
c. hypothalamus
d. a neuromuscular junction

5.2   Which of the following carries nerve impulses towards the cell body of a neuron?
a. axons
b. nodes of Ranvier
c. myelin
d. dendrons

5.3   Which of the following statements is *false?*
a. Sensory nerve fibres carry information towards the central nervous system.
b. Most nerve fibres within the grey matter of the brain are myelinated.
c. A ganglion is a collection of nerve cell bodies.
d. The autonomic nervous system consists mainly of visceral motor nerves.

5.4   The pons, medulla and cerebellum together form the —
a. forebrain
b. midbrain
c. hindbrain
d. cerebral hemispheres

5.5   Working from the outer surface of the brain to the inside, the meningeal layers are:
a. pia mater, arachnoid mater, dura mater
b. dura mater, arachnoid mater, pia mater
c. arachnoid mater, dura mater, pia mater
d. dura mater, pia mater, arachnoid mater

5.6   The aqueduct of Silvius lies within which part of the central nervous system?
a. midbrain
b. hindbrain
c. spinal cord
d. forebrain

5.7   Which of the following cranial nerves is responsible for gustation?
a. olfactory
b. glossopharyngeal
c. optic
d. trochlear

5.8   Which of the following statements is *true?*
a. The photoreceptor cells within the back of the eye and known as rods are responsible for colour vision.
b. The pupil of the cat is rounded.
c. Aqueous humour lies within the posterior chamber of the eye.
d. The cells of the tapetum lucidum reflect light back to the photoreceptor cells of the retina.

5.9   Which of the following reflexes is routinely used to test for the level of anaesthesia?
a. palpebral
b. panniculus
c. anal
d. patella

5.10 Which structure is used to monitor balance?
a. organ of corti
b. tympanic membrane
c. malleus
d. utricle and saccule

6. The Endocrine System

6.1 The chemical messengers sent out by the organs of the endocrine system are:
   a. glucose
   b. enzymes
   c. hormones
   d. nerve impulses

6.2 Which of the following statements is *false?* Endocrine glands:
   a. may be controlled by levels of chemicals or other hormones in the blood
   b. secrete hormones directly into their target organs by means of a duct
   c. secrete hormones that are designed to specifically affect the target organ and no other
   d. secrete hormones directly into the bloodstream

6.3 Which of the following are classed as endocrine glands?
   a. ovary
   b. pancreas
   c. thyroid gland
   d. all of the above

6.4 Which of the following hormones is secreted by the posterior pituitary?
   a. ACTH
   b. TSH
   c. ADH
   d. FSH

6.5 Which of the following hormones has an effect on the kidney?
   a. ADH
   b. oxytocin
   c. TSH
   d. calcitonin

6.6 Which of the following is *not* secreted by the adrenal cortex?
   a. aldosterone
   b. cortisol
   c. oestrogen
   d. adrenaline

6.7 When an animal is very frightened and likely to attack you, which of the following is happening inside the animal?
   a. salivary secretion increases so the animal dribbles
   b. blood glucose levels rise
   c. respiratory rate slows down
   d. levels of cortisol and corticosterone in the blood decrease

6.8 Polydipsia, polyuria, polyphagia and bilateral symmetrical alopecia are symptoms of:
   a. diabetes mellitus
   b. diabetes insipidus
   c. Addison's disease
   d. Cushing's disease

6.9 Testosterone is secreted by which cells?
   a. islets of Langerhans
   b. sertoli cells
   c. Brunner's glands
   d. cells of Leydig

6.10 Hypoglycaemia or lowered blood glucose will stimulate the secretion of which pancreatic hormone?
   a. glucagon
   b. insulin
   c. antidiuretic hormone
   d. somatostatin

7. The Blood Vascular System

7.1   Which of the following statements is *true*?
a. Blood entering the right atrium is well oxygenated.
b. The right ventricle pumps blood into the systemic circulation via the pulmonary vein.
c. Blood returning to the heart enters the left atrium via the cranial and caudal venae cavae.
d. The right ventricle pumps blood into the pulmonary circulation via the pulmonary artery.

7.2   Which branch of the aorta transports oxygenated blood to the kidneys?
a. renal vein
b. hepatic artery
c. renal artery
d. hepatic portal vein

7.3   The fibrous threads that attach the mitral valve to the papillary muscle of the ventricular wall are known as:
a. Purkinje fibres
b. chordae tendinae
c. bundle of His
d. collateral ligaments

7.4   Which granulocyte produces histamine?
a. basophil
b. eosinophil
c. neutrophil
d. macrophage

7.5   Which of the following are essential to the blood clotting mechanism?
a. potassium and vitamin D
b. calcium and vitamin K
c. sodium and vitamin C
d. iron and vitamin B

7.6   The area of modified cardiac muscle cells in the wall of the right atrium that initiates the heartbeat is referred to as the:
a. atrioventricular node
b. Purkinje fibres
c. bundle of His
d. sinoatrial node

7.7   In the foetal circulation, the shunt that connects the pulmonary artery and aorta is called the —
a. ductus venosus
b. foramen ovale
c. ductus arteriosus
d. falciform ligament

7.8   What is the name of the main lymphatic duct that arises in the abdomen?
a. tracheal duct
b. cisterna chyli
c. right lymphatic duct
d. cisterna magna

7.9   Which of the following is *not* a function of the spleen?
a. production of thrombocytes
b. storage of blood
c. destruction of worn out red blood cells
d. production of lymphocytes

7.10 Which of the following cells is involved in the humoral immune response?
a. macrophage
b. B-lymphocyte
c. neutrophil
d. T-lymphocyte

8. The Respiratory System

8.1   What prevents food from entering the nasal
       chamber when an animal swallows?
       a. nasal septum
       b. soft palate
       c. epiglottis
       d. nasal conchae

8.2   Which part of the respiratory system is also
       responsible for the production of sound?
       a. hyoid apparatus
       b. eustachian tube
       c. pharynx
       d. larynx

8.3   Which type of epithelium lines the trachea?
       a. ciliated columnar
       b. simple squamous
       c. stratified squamous
       d. transitional

8.4   Which of the following statements is *true?* The
       route taken by the inspired air from the
       pharynx into the lungs is —
       a. trachea, larynx, bronchi, bronchioles, alveolar
           ducts, alveolar sacs
       b. larynx, bronchi, trachea, bronchioles, alveolar
           sacs, alveolar ducts
       c. larynx, trachea, bronchioles, bronchi, alveolar
           sacs, alveolar ducts
       d. larynx, trachea, bronchi, bronchioles, alveolar
           ducts, alveolar sacs

8.5   Where does gaseous exchange take place in the
       respiratory system?
       a. bronchioles, alveolar ducts and alveoli
       b. alveoli only
       c. respiratory bronchioles only
       d. alveolar ducts and alveoli

8.6   What is the fourth lobe of the right lung of a
       dog called?
       a. apical lobe
       b. cardiac lobe
       c. the right lung does not have a fourth lobe
       d. accessory lobe

8.7   Which muscle is responsible for increasing the
       volume of the thoracic cavity during
       inspiration?
       a. diaphragm
       b. hypaxial
       c. external oblique
       d. epaxial

8.8   Which reflex prevents over inflation of the
       lungs?
       a. Howell-Joly
       b. Hering-Breuer
       c. cough
       d. Flehman's

8.9   The chemoreceptors that monitor oxygen levels
       and the pH of the blood are located in the —
       a. bronchi and bronchioles
       b. alveoli
       c. aortic and carotid bodies
       d. jugular vein

8.10   The air left in the airways and lungs after a
       forced expiration is referred to as the:
       a. residual volume
       b. dead space
       c. vital capacity
       d. tidal volume

9. The Digestive System

9.1   The process of breaking food down into small soluble units is known as:
    a. ingestion
    b. digestion
    c. absorption
    d. excretion

9.2   The cleft in the upper lip is known as the:
    a. soft palate
    b. carnassial
    c. philtrum
    d. tubercle

9.3   The formula for the deciduous dentition in the cat is:
    a. $[I3/3, C 1/1, PM 3/2] \times 2 = 26$
    b. $[I3/3, C1/1, PM 3/3] \times 2 = 28$
    c. $[I3/3, C1/1, PM 4/4, M 2/3] \times 2 = 42$
    d. $[I3/3, C1/1, PM 3/2, M 1/1] \times 2 = 30$

9.4   Which of the following is *not* part of the small intestine?
    a. stomach
    b. duodenum
    c. jejunum
    d. ileum

9.5   Food passes through the parts of the large intestine in which order?
    a. ascending colon, descending colon, transverse colon, caecum, rectum
    b. descending colon, transverse colon, ascending colon, rectum, caecum
    c. caecum, ascending colon, descending colon, transverse colon, rectum
    d. caecum, ascending colon, transverse colon, descending colon, rectum

9.6   The chief cells in the gastric mucosa produce which part of the gastric juices?
    a. pepsin
    b. pepsinogen
    c. hydrochloric acid
    d. mucus

9.7   Which salivary gland lies within the orbit of the skull?
    a. parotid
    b. sublingual
    c. mandibular
    d. zygomatic

9.8   Food resulting from digestion in the stomach is:
    a. chyme with an acid pH
    b. chyle with a neutral pH
    c. chyme with an alkaline pH
    d. bile with a neutral pH

9.9   Which of the following is *not* a function of the liver?
    a. production of plasma proteins
    b. storage of iron
    c. regulation of fluid volume in the fluid compartments
    d. formation of red blood cells in the foetus

9.10 Amino acids resulting from the digestion of protein are carried to the liver by the:
    a. lacteals
    b. hepatic portal vein
    c. hepatic vein
    d. hepatic artery

10. The Urinary System

10.1 Which of the following statements is *false*?
  a. The position of the kidney in the abdomen is described as being retroperitoneal.
  b. The right kidney is caudal to the left kidney.
  c. The kidneys lie in the cranial abdomen closely attached to the lumbar hypaxial muscles.
  d. The ovaries and the adrenal glands lie close to the cranial pole of each kidney.

10.2 The basin shaped structure in the centre of the kidney is called the:
  a. cortex
  b. hilus
  c. pelvis
  d. medulla

10.3 The loop of Henle of each nephron:
  a. lies within the medulla and is lined with simple squamous epithelium
  b. lies in the cortex and is lined with cuboidal epithelium
  c. lies in the medulla and is lined with columnar epithelium
  d. lies in the kidney pyramids and collects urine from several nephrons

10.4 Which of the following does *not* occur in the proximal convoluted tubule?
  a. secretion of penicillin
  b. reabsorption of glucose
  c. control of acid/base balance
  d. reabsorption of water

10.5 Which of the following statements is *false*?
  a. Aldosterone is secreted by the anterior pituitary gland at the base of the brain.
  b. Aldosterone acts mainly on the distal convoluted tubules and controls the reabsorption of sodium.
  c. ADH is secreted when an animal is dehydrated.
  d. The release of aldosterone is stimulated by angiotensin.

10.6 Which of the following hormones does *not* have an effect on the kidney?
  a. renin
  b. aldosterone
  c. antidiuretic hormone
  d. erythropoietin

10.7 If an animal is over-hydrated which of the following will happen?
  a. Blood pressure will fall and will be detected by baroreceptors in the blood vessel walls.
  b. Osmotic pressure will rise and the osmoreceptors will stimulate the thirst centre.
  c. Secretion of ADH will decrease and a large volume of dilute urine will be excreted.
  d. Water will be resorbed into the capillaries of the medulla from the loops of Henle.

10.8 If an animal is fed on a high salt diet which of the following will *not* happen?
  a. The osmotic pressure of the blood will increase.
  b. Water will be drawn into the circulation by osmosis, increasing the circulating blood volume.
  c. The animal will become hypertensive.
  d. Aldosterone secretion will rise and sodium will be resorbed from the distal convoluted tubules.

10.9 The bladder is lined by which type of epithelium?
  a. squamous
  b. ciliated columnar
  c. transitional
  d. cuboidal

10.10 Normal urine contains:
  a. glucose, water and urea
  b. water, salts and urea
  c. protein, amino acids and water
  d. urea, crystals and glucose

11. The Reproductive System

11.1 Which of the following is *not* a function of the male reproductive tract?
a. secretion of hormones to produce the secondary sexual characteristics
b. transportation of urine from the bladder to the outside of the body
c. production of fluids to wash the sperm into the female tract
d. production of sperm to fertilise the ova of the female

11.2 At what age would you expect to find the testes in the scrotum of the dog?
a. 12 weeks post-partum
b. 35 weeks of gestation
c. just prior to parturition
d. 6 months post-partum

11.3 Which of the following are seen in the cat and *not* in the dog?
a. bulbourethral glands
b. preprostatic urethra
c. barbed glans penis
d. all of the above

11.4 The os penis of the dog lies:
a. ventral to the urethra
b. dorsal to the urethra
c. caudal to the prostate
d. in the centre of the urethra

11.5 Spermatozoa are produced:
a. by mitosis and contain the diploid number of chromosomes
b. by meiosis and contain the haploid number of chromosomes
c. by binary fission and contain the haploid number of chromosomes
d. by meiosis and contain the diploid number of chromosomes

11.6 The bitch and the queen are described as:
a. primigravid
b. uniparous
c. multigravid
d. multiparous

11.7 Pseudocyesis is better known as:
a. pregnancy
b. fertilisation
c. false pregnancy
d. ovulation

11.8 The fold of peritoneum supporting the uterus within the peritoneal cavity is the:
a. broad ligament
b. mesosalpinx
c. mesovarium
d. mesocolon

11.9 The queen is described as being:
a. a spontaneous ovulator and seasonally polyoestrous
b. an induced ovulator and monoestrous
c. an induced ovulator and seasonally polyoestrous
d. a spontaneous ovulator and monoestrous

11.10 Within the inner cell mass of the developing embryo the ectoderm forms:
a. the lining of the digestive tract
b. the trophoblast
c. the skin and nervous system
d. the musculoskeletal system

12. The Common Integument

12.1 In which layer of the epidermis are new cells manufactured?
  a. stratum granulosum
  b. stratum germinativum
  c. stratum lucidum
  d. stratum corneum

12.2 In which layer of the skin are the sensory nerve endings found?
  a. hypodermis
  b. epidermis
  c. dermis
  d. subcutis

12.3 Where do the ducts of the sebaceous glands open into?
  a. the surface layer of the epithelium
  b. the hair follicle
  c. the sweat glands
  d. the hypodermis

12.4 Where are ceruminous glands found?
  a. opening onto the eyelids
  b. around the circumference of the anus
  c. associated with each hair follicle
  d. in the external ear canal

12.5 Which of the following statements is the most accurate?
  a. Each hair follicle contains one guard hair and several wool hairs.
  b. Each hair follicle contains a wool hair only.
  c. Each hair follicle contains one wool hair and several guard hairs.
  d. Each hair follicle contains several guard hairs and many wool hairs.

12.6 How many pads are found on the hind paw of the dog?
  a. 7
  b. 4
  c. 5
  d. 6

12.7. Which muscle unsheathes the claws of a cat?
  a. digital extensor muscle
  b. digital flexor muscle
  c. carpal flexor muscle
  d. carpal extensor muscle

12.8 Which part of the distal phalanx is covered by the claw?
  a. anconeal process
  b. sole
  c. ungual process
  d. claw fold

12.9 Where are sudoriferous glands found in the dog?
  a. at the base of the tail
  b. on the nose and foot pads
  c. associated with each hair follicle
  d. in the ear canal

12.10 Which of the following is *not* a function of the integument?
  a secretion of pheromones
  b. production of vitamin E
  c. protection from invasion by bacteria
  d. thermoregulation

SECTION 2 – EXOTIC SPECIES

13. Birds

13.1 Which of the following characteristics is possessed only by the class Aves?
a. ability to fly
b. feathers
c. ability to lay eggs
d. warm-blooded

13.2 The sternum of the bird is extended into a flattened:
a. coracoid
b. quadrate
c. keel
d. pygostyle

13.3 Which of the following statements is *false?*
a. Some of the bones of the skeleton are filled with sacs full of air to reduce the weight.
b. There are always seven cervical vertebrae in the neck no matter how long the neck.
c. At the base of the tail is a preen gland whose secretions are vital for the health of the feathers.
d. There is no diaphragm to divide the body cavity into thorax and abdomen.

13.4 The feathers attached to the ulna of the wing are the:
a. contour feathers
b. filoplume
c. primaries
d. secondaries

13.5 Which is the most developed special sense in the bird?
a. sight
b. touch
c. smell
d. taste

13.6 Which of the following statements is *false?*
a. Air passes through the lungs twice – the second passage is the most efficient.
b. Many thin-walled air sacs lead out of the lungs and occupy most of the body cavity.
c. The lungs are large, flexible and spongy and lie close to the ventral body wall.
d. There is no diaphragm separating the thorax from the abdomen.

13.7 The passage of food down the digestive tract is:
a. crop, proventriculus, gizzard, duodenum, jejunum
b. oesophagus, stomach, duodenum, jejeunum
c. gizzard, proventriculus, crop, duodenum, ileum
d. oesophagus, crop, gizzard, proventriculus

13.8 In the bird, the principal excretory product is:
a. urea
b. ammonia
c. urates
d. bile

13.9 Which part of the female reproductive tract is responsible for the addition of albumen to the bird's egg?
a. magnum
b. isthmus
c. shell gland
d. vagina

13.10 By which method could you identify the sex of a budgerigar?
a. DNA testing
b. surgical sexing
c. sexual dimorphism
d. by listening to the birdsong

14. Mammals

14.1 Members of the order Lagomorpha can be distinguished from members of the order Rodentia by examination of:
a. ears
b. genitalia
c. teeth
d. cheek muscles

14.2 The digestive tract of the rabbit and the herbivorous rodent has an enlarged:
a. stomach
b. spleen
c. jejunum
d. caecum

14.3 The dental formula of the rabbit is:
a. I1/1, C0/0, PM0/0, M 3/3 × 2 = 16
b. I2/1, C0/0, PM3/2, M 3/3 × 2 = 28
c. I1/1, C0/0, PM1/1, M 3/3 × 2 = 20
d. I3/3, C1/1, PM3/3, M 1/2 × 2 = 34

14.4 The space between the incisors and the cheek teeth of rabbits and rodents is known as the:
a. diastema
b. philtrum
c. dewlap
d. acromion

14.5 Young that are born blind, deaf, hairless and totally dependent on the mother are described as being:
a. precocial
b. nidicolous
c. altricial
d. nidifugous

14.6 Which of the following species gives birth to precocial young?
a. *Mustela putorius furo*
b. *Oryctolagus cuniculus*
c. *Mus musculus*
d. *Chinchilla lanigera*

14.7 Which of the following species is an induced ovulator?
a. the ferret
b. the mouse
c. the guinea pig
d. the chipmunk

14.8 Which of the following statements is *false?*
a. Jill ferrets can suffer from a fatal anemia if not allowed to breed at regular intervals.
b. The jill is a spontaneous ovulator and ovulation occurs on the tenth day of the season.
c. Ferrets are true carnivores and belong to the family Mustelidae.
d. The male ferret has a J-shaped os penis which lies in the caudal portion of the penis.

14.9 The males of which of the following species have teats on the ventral body wall?
a. *Rattus norvegicus*
b. *Tamias sibiricus*
c. *Cavia porcellus*
d. *Mesocricetus auratus*

14.10 The gestation period of the chinchilla is:
a. 111 days
b. 9 weeks
c. 28–32 days
d. 15–18 days

15. Reptiles and Fish

15.1 Tortoises and terrapins belong to the order:
a. Rhyncocephalia
b. Crocodilia
c. Chelonia
d. Squamata

15.2 Which of the following statements is *false?*
a. The body cavity of the reptile is not divided into two by a diaphragm.
b. In the peripheral circulation of the reptile a renal portal system transports blood from the hindlimbs and tail directly to the kidney.
c. Reptiles do not possess a bladder for the storage of urine.
d. Reptiles may be oviparous (egg layers) or oviviparous (live bearers).

15.3 The sex of a tortoise can be determined by examining:
a. the tail length – males have longer tails
b. the plastron – that of the female is convex and of the male is concave
c. the caudal scute – in the female it may curve upwards
d. all of the above

15.4 The ability of some species of lizard to shed the tail and grow a new one is known as:
a. ecdysis
b. autotomy
c. caecotrophy
d. mutation

15.5 Jacobsen's organ, located in the mouth of some reptiles, is associated with which sense?
a. smell
b. sight
c. hearing
d. touch

15.6 Which one of the following statements is *false?*
a. Snakes do not have eyelids but have a transparent spectacle over the eye.
b. Some snakes show evidence of vestigial legs.
c. All species of snake have external ears which they use to detect their prey.
d. Some snakes lay eggs while others bear live young.

15.7 Which body system does not open into the cloaca of the snake?
a. digestive
b. urinary
c. reproductive
d. circulatory

15.8. In fish a physostomous swim bladder is refilled with air by:
a. a gas gland lying in the wall of the bladder
b. swimming to the surface and taking a mouthful of air
c. excretory gases formed by the gut
d. descending to the bottom and increasing the air pressure

15.9 The ability of shoals of fish to move simultaneously is thought to be linked to the presence of:
a. the lateral line
b. chromatophores in the skin which change colour
c. the presence of the glycocalyx which reduces friction
d. coordinated movements of the tail fins

15.10. The function of the gill rakers projecting from the gill arches is to:
a. extract oxygen from the water passing over them
b. prevent damage to the gills by food particles taken into the mouth cavity
c. prevent damage to the gills from objects in the water
d. support the gill arches

MULTIPLE CHOICE ANSWERS

1.1 c	3.6 c	6.1 c	8.6 d	11.1 b	13.6 c
1.2 a	3.7 d	6.2 b	8.7 a	11.2 a	13.7 a
1.3 b	3.8 b	6.3 d	8.8 b	11.3 d	13.8 c
1.4 b	3.9 a	6.4 c	8.9 c	11.4 b	13.9 a
1.5 c	3.10 b	6.5 a	8.10 a	11.5 b	13.10 c
1.6 b		6.6 d		11.6 d	
1.7 a	4.1 b	6.7 b	9.1 b	11.7 c	14.1 c
1.8 a	4.2 c	6.8 d	9.2 c	11.8 a	14.2 d
1.9 b	4.3 a	6.9 d	9.3 a	11.9 c	14.3 b
1.10 c	4.4 d	6.10 a	9.4 a	11.10 c	14.4 a
	4.5 b		9.5 d		14.5 c
2.1 c	4.6 c	7.1 d	9.6 b	12.1 b	14.6 d
2.2 d	4.7 a	7.2 c	9.7 d	12.2 c	14.7 a
2.3 c	4.8 d	7.3 b	9.8 a	12.3 b	14.8 b
2.4 c	4.9 c	7.4 a	9.9 c	12.4 d	14.9 c
2.5 b	4.10 a	7.5 b	9.10 b	12.5 a	14.10 a
2.6 c		7.6 d		12.6 c	
2.7 d	5.1 c	7.7 c	10.1 b	12.7 b	15.1 c
2.8 a	5.2 d	7.8 b	10.2 c	12.8 c	15.2 c
2.9 b	5.3 b	7.9 a	10.3 a	12.9 b	15.3 d
2.10 c	5.4 c	7.10 b	10.4 c	12.10 b	15.4 b
	5.5 b		10.5 a		15.5 a
3.1 c	5.6 a	8.1 b	10.6 d	13.1 b	15.6 c
3.2 a	5.7 b	8.2 d	10.7 c	13.2 c	15.7 d
3.3 d	5.8 d	8.3 a	10.8 d	13.3 b	15.8 b
3.4 c	5.9 a	8.4 d	10.9 c	13.4 d	15.9 a
3.5 b	5.10 d	8.5 b	10.10 b	13.5 a	15.10 b

INDEX

Page numbers in *italic* indicate a figure. Entries refer to the dog and the cat except where otherwise indicated.

abdominal cavity 24–5, *24, 26*
abdominal muscles 49–50, *50*
abdominal viscera 24
abduction, of a limb 42
absorption of food, small intestine 107, 118
acetabulum 39
acetyl choline 56, 57
Achilles tendon 54
acids in the body 13
    and bases (alkalis) 14
ACTH (adrenocorticotrophic hormone) 78, 79
actin (thin) filaments 45, *45*
active transport mechanisms (cell membrane) 6
adduction, of a limb 42
adductor muscles 52, *53*
adenohypophysis 79, *82*
adipose (fatty) tissue 19, 20
ADP (adenosine diphosphate) 7, *7*
adrenal cortex 79, 82
adrenal glands 77, *77*, 79, 82–3, 122, *123*
adrenal hormones 79
adrenal medulla 79, 82–3
adrenal sex hormones 79, 82
adrenaline (epinephrine) 56, 79, 82–3
adrenocorticotrophic hormone (ACTH) 78, 79
afferent nerves 59
agranulocytes (agranular leucocytes) 85, *85*, 86, 87
alar fold 98, *98*
albumin 85
aldosterone 82
alkalis and acids 14
altricial young, rabbit 178
alveoli 101–2, *102*
amino acids 14, *15*, 118
aminopeptidase 118
amphiarthroses 42
Amphibia (class) 3
amylases 118
anabolic reactions 15
anaesthetics, for birds 168
anal sacs
    impacted 119
    scent marking 119
anal sphincter 119
anaphase of mitosis 9, *9*
anaphase I of meiosis *10*, 11
anaphase II of meiosis *10*, 11
anastomosis 91
anatomical definitions 4–5, *4*
anatomy (definition) 3
animal classification (taxonomy) 3–4
animal kingdom (classification) 3

anions 13
annulus fibrosus 33, *34*
anterior (or cranial) (definition) 4, *4*
anterior chamber 69, 71
anterior pituitary gland 79, *82*
anterior tibialis muscle 54, *54*
antibodies 85, 87, 96
anticoagulants 87
antidiuretic hormone (ADH) 78, 80
antigens 96
antiperistalsis 113, 119
anus 107, *107, 108*
aorta 88, *89*, 91, *92*
aortic valve 88, *89*
aponeurosis 46
    linea alba 49–50, *50*
appendicular skeleton 36–41
aqueous humour 71
arachnoid mater 62, *62*
areolar tissue (loose connective tissue) 19, 20, *20*
arterial circulation 91, *92*
arteries *90*, 90–1
arterioles 91
asternal ('false') ribs 35, *36*
atlas (first cervical vertebra) *27*, 30, 34
atoms 13
ATP (adenosine triphosphate) and energy 6, 7, *7*, 15, 45
atria 88, 89
atrioventricular node *89*, 90
atrioventricular valves 88, *89*
atrophy of muscles 46
auditory ossicles 73, *74*, 75
automatic reflexes 66
autonomic nervous system 60, 66, *67, 68*
Aves (birds) 3 *see also* birds
axis 34, *35*
axon hillock 56
axons 23, *23*, 56, *57*
azygous vein *92*, 93

backbone
    animals with 3
    animals without 3
balance
    and coordination, cerebellum 61
    while in motion 75
    while standing still 75
balanitis (balanoprosthitis) 139
ball and socket joints 44
'barium meal' X-rays 113, *114*
bases (alkalis)
    and acids 14
    in the body 13
basophils 85, *86*, 87
beak 159, 170, *170*
bicarbonate ions 13, 85
biceps brachii muscle 51, *51, 52*
biceps femoris muscle 52, *53*
bicuspid valve 88, *89*
bilaterally cryptorchid 137
bile 116, 119

bile canaliculi 119, 120
bile duct 116, 119, *120*
bile salts 116, 117, 118
bilirubin 86, 116
binary fission 8
binocular vision (3D) 68, *69*
bipolar neurons *70*, 71
birds 159–72
    anaesthetising 168
    bone structure 159, *160*
    brain 164, *164*
    circulatory system 168, 168–9
    crop 169, *170*
    differences in beak shape 170, *170*
    digestive system 169, 169–70
    droppings 170, *172*
    egg formation 171–2
    erythrocytes (red blood cells) 169
    eyesight 164, 164–5
    feather structure 161, *163*
    flight muscles 159
    gizzard 169, 170
    handling 163
    hearing 165
    heart 168
    intubation of 167
    leg and foot *160*, 160–1, *161*
    moulting 162
    perching reflex 161
    reproductive system *171*, 171–2
    respiration *167*, 167–8
    respiratory system 165–8, *166*
    salivary glands 170
    sense of smell 165
    sense of taste 165
    sense of touch 165
    sex of offspring 172
    sexual differentiation 172
    skeletal modifications 159–61, *160*
    skeleton 159–61, *160*
    skull 159–60, *161*
    splanchnic bones around the eye 41
    types and functions of feathers 161–2, *163*
    urinary system 170, *171*
    wing structure *160*, 161, *162*
biting action 108
bladder (urinary) 25, *26*, 122, *123*, 131
blind spot 69, 71
blink reflex 72
blood
    cells 1, 11, 85, *85*
    composition 84–7, *85*
    regulation functions 84
    specialised connective tissue 19
    transport functions 84
blood–brain barrier 62
blood circulation, in the fetus 93
blood clotting 84, 96
    cascade mechanism 87
    factors affecting 87

blood glucose levels 119
  control of 81, *81*
blood pressure 84, 90
  and osmoregulation 128–30, *129, 130*
blood vascular system 11, 84–97
blood vessels, types and functions *90,* 90–1
blood volume 84
B-lymphocytes 87
body, basic plan 5
body cavities 5, 23–6
body chemistry 11–15
body covering (integument) 5
body structures, terms used to describe 4, 4–5
body systems 5, 17
bone marrow 27
  production of granulocytes 86
  production of lymphocytes 87
  production of platelets 87
  production of red blood cells 85, 86
bones 19, 20–1, *21*
  categories by shape 27–8, *28*
  development of 28, *29*
  flat 27
  irregular 28
  long 27, *28,* 28, 29
  of birds 159, *160*
  of the forelimb *27,* 36–9
  of the hindlimb 39–41
  of the oral cavity 108
  pneumatic 28
  sesamoid 28
  short 27–8
  splanchnic 28
  structure and function 27–8
bony labyrinth *74,* 74
brachial plexus 65
brachialis muscle 51, *51*
brachiocephalicus muscle 51
brachycephalic skull shape 32, *33*
brain 59
  of birds 164, *164*
  protection of 61–2
  structures and functions 60–1, *60, 61*
breathing, mechanics of 104–5
bronchi 101, *101*
bronchioles 101, *101*
Brunner's glands 116, 118
bulbourethral glands, cat 139
bundle of His fibres *89,* 90
bursa 46, *47*
  on the Achilles tendon 54

caecotrophs 176–7
caecum 107, *107, 108,* 118
caesarean section, rabbit 177
calcaneus 40, *41, 43*
calcitonin 78, 80, *80*
calcium 13, 14, 85
  and blood clotting 87
  and muscle contraction 45
  and transmission of nerve impulses 57
cancellous (spongy) bone 21
canine teeth *110,* 110–11
capillaries *90,* 91
capillary beds 91
carbohydrates (polysaccharides) 14, *14*
  digestion of 108, 116–18
  in food 116
  metabolism, in the liver 119

carbon compounds 14–15
cardiac muscle 22–3, *22,* 89
cardiac sphincter 113, 114, *115*
cardiovascular system 5
carnassial teeth *110,* 110–11
carnivores 4
  teeth 109–10
carpal bones 38, *38*
carpal extensor muscles 51, *52*
carpal flexor muscles *52,* 52
carpus 38, *38*
carrier proteins 6
cartilage 19, 20, *21*
cartilaginous joints 41, 42
cat
  classification of 3
  clavicle 36
  endocrine glands *77, 77*
  humerus *37, 38*
  os penis 28, 41
  scapula *175*
  skull shapes 31
catabolic reactions 15
cataracts 71
cations 13
cauda equina 63, *64*
caudal (definition) 4, *4*
caudal (coccygeal) vertebrae *27,* 32
  shapes of 34, *35*
caudal vena cava 88, *89, 92,* 93, 119
cavernous erectile tissue 137, *138*
cell body (neuron) 56, *57*
cell membrane 5–6, *6,* 7–8
cells 5–15
  bathed in interstitial fluid 11
  division 7, 8–11
  energy supply 6
  in tissues 17–18
  organelles 5, *6,* 7–8
  structure and function 5–8, *6*
cells of Leydig (interstitial cells) 81, 135
cellular immune response 87, 96
central nervous system (CNS) 56, 59–63
centrioles *6,* 7, 8–9
centromere 9
centrosome 5, *6,* 7
cerebellar hypoplasia 61
cerebellum *60,* 61, *61*
cerebral cortex (grey matter) 60
cerebrospinal fluid (CSF) 11, 60, 61
  collecting samples 61
cerebrum (cerebral hemispheres) 60, *60, 61*
ceruminous glands 73
cervical vertebrae *27,* 32
  shapes of 34, *35*
cervix *140,* 140–1
Cetaceans 4
cheeks 108
Chelonians (tortoises, turtles, terrapins) 191–3
  cardiovascular system 191
  digestive system 191, *192, 193*
  respiratory system 191, *193*
  sexual differentiation 192–3, *193*
  shell 191, *192*
  skeleton 191, *192*
  urogenital system 192, *192, 193*
chemical transmitter substances 56
chemistry of the body 11–15
chemoreceptors, respiration control 105

chinchilla (*Chinchilla laniger*) 178
  dentition 183
  diet 184
  digestive system 183
  morphology 183
  physiological and behavioural data 188
  reproductive data 189
  reproductive system 184
  sexual differentiation 184
chipmunk (*Tamias sibiricus*) 178
  digestive system 181
  morphology 180–1
  physiological and behavioural data 188
  reproductive data 189
  reproductive system 181
chloride 13, 84
cholinesterases 57
chorionic gonadotrophin 79
choroid 70
choroid plexuses 61
chromatids 9
chromosomes 7
  changes during mitosis 8–9, *9*
  'crossing over' 11
  diploid number 8
  haploid number 8, 10, 11
chyle 116, *117,* 118
chyme 115, 118
cilia 6, 7–8
ciliary body 69, 70, 71
ciliary muscle 69, 70, 71
ciliated epithelium 17, 18
ciliated mucous epithelium 30
  in the trachea 100–1
  inside the nose 98
circulatory system 90–3
  in birds 168, 168–9
circumduction, of an extremity 42
cisterna chyli 94, *94, 96,* 116, 118
class (classification) 3
classification system 3–4
clavicle 36
claws 38, 39, 155–6, *156*
clitoris *140,* 142
collagen 15
collagen fibres 20, *20*
collateral ligaments 42, *43*
collecting duct (nephron) 124, *125*
  functions of *127,* 128
colon 107, *107, 108*
  functions of 118
colostrum 143
columnar cells 17, 18
common bile duct 116
common integument 151–6
compact bone 21
compounds 13
concentration gradient 6
conchae 98, *99*
conditional reflex 66
condylar joints 44
condyle 29
cones (light sensitive cells) 70, 71
conjunctiva 69, 69
connective tissue 17
  types and functions 18–21
coordinating systems of the body 5
copper 14
coprophagia, rodents 176–7, 180, 182, 183
cornea 69, 69, 72
coronary veins 92, 93

corpus callosum 60
corpus luteum *141*, 143
corticosteroids 82
corticosterone 82
cortisol 82
costal arch 35, *36*
costal cartilage 35, *36*
cough reflex 101
    absent in reptiles 191
cow
    milk fever 57
    os cordis 41
cranial (definition) 4, *4*
cranial nerves *61*, 63, 65
cranial vena cava 88, *89*, 92, *92*
cranium 29–30
cremaster muscle 137
crop, in birds *169*, 170
cruciate ligaments 42, *43*
cryptorchidism 137
crypts of Lieberkuhn 116, 118
cuboidal cells *17*, 18
Cushing's disease 82
cytoplasm 5, *6*, 7

Dartos muscle 135, 137
daughter cells, produced by mitosis 9,
    9
dead space, in the respiratory tract
    101, 105
deciduous dentition 110–11
deep (definition) 4
defaecation 119
deferent duct (vas deferens, ductus
    deferens) *134*, *135*, 137
deglutition (swallowing) *112*,
    112–13
dehydration 13
    signs of 128–9
dendrites 56, 57
dendrons 23, *23*, 56, *57*
dense connective tissue 19, *20*
dental arches 109
dental formulae 110
dentition
    deciduous 110–11
    permanent 110–11
dermis 152, *152*
dew claw 38, *38*, 39, 40, *41*
diabetes mellitus 81, 127
diaphragm 24, *24*, *25*, 104–5
    absent in reptiles 191
    structure of 49, *49*
diaphysis (shaft) of a bone 28, *29*
diarrhoea 119
diarthroses 42
diastole 89, 90
diffusion 11–12, *12*
    across a cell membrane 6
digastricus muscle 47, *47*
digestion 107, 116–18
digestive enzymes 15
digestive juices 11, 117
digestive system 5, 24–5, 107–21
    accessory glands 107
    barium X-ray series 113, *114*
    birds *169*, 169–70
    parts of 107, *107*, *108*
digital extensor muscles 51, *52*, 54,
    54
digital flexor muscles *52*, 52, 54, *54*
digits 38, *38*
dipeptides 14
distal (definition) 4, 5

distal convoluted tubule 124, *125*
    functions of *127*, 128
distichiasis 72
diuretics 128
DNA (deoxyribonucleic acid) 7, 8
dog
    classification of 3
    clavicle 36
    digestive system *107*
    eclampsia in bitches 57
    elbow dysplasia 37
    femur *40*
    hip dysplasia 39, 54
    humerus 37, *38*
    hyoid apparatus 32
    mandible (medial and lateral
        views) *30*
    nose 98
    os penis 28, 41
    pelvis 39
    radius and ulna 37, *38*
    ribcage *36*
    ribs *36*
    scapula *36*
    skeleton 27
    skull *30*
    skull shapes 31–2, *33*
    tarsus *41*
    tibia and fibula *40*
    upper respiratory tract *99*
dolichocephalic skull shape 32, *33*
domestic cat *see* cat
domestic dog *see* dog
dopamine 56
dorsal (definition) 4, *4*
ductus arteriosus 93
ductus venosus 93
duodenum 107, *107*, *108*, 116
dura mater 62, *62*
dwarfism 80

ear, hearing and balance 73–5
ecdysis
    lizards 194
    reptiles 191
    snakes 197
eclampsia in bitches 57
ectropion 72
efferent nerves 59
egg (bird), formation of 171–2
ejaculation 137
elastic cartilage 20
elastic fibres 20, *20*
elastin 15
elbow (olecranon) 37, *38*
elbow dysplasia in dogs 37
elbow joint 37, *43*
elbow region, muscles of 51, *52*
electrolyte 13
elements 13
embolus (clot) 87
embryo and fetus 146–9
    development of the embryo *148*,
        149
    development of the fetus 149
    developmental terminology 146
    endochondral ossification 28, *29*
    extra-embryonic membranes
        147–9, *148*
    fertilisation and cell division
        146–7, *147*, *148*
    fetal blood circulation 93
    germ cell layers 147, *148*
    neural tube 59

placenta 149
endochondral ossification 20, 28, *29*
endocrine glands 18, 77, *77*
    associated hormones 78–9
endocrine system 5, 60, 77–83
    functions 77
endocytosis 7, 8, *8*
endolymph 74, *74*, 75, *75*
endoplasmic reticulum (ER)
    rough 5, *6*, 7
    smooth 5, *6*, 7
endothelium 17, 24–5
energy
    role of mitochondria 7, *7*
    supply in the cell 6
    use in the body, metabolism 15
enterokinase 118
entropion 72
enzymes 15, 116–17
    as catalysts 15
    for digestion 117–18
    transport of 84
eosinophils 85, *86*, 86–7
epaxial muscles 48, *48*
epicondyle 29
epidermis 151–2, *152*
    thickness of 153
epididymis *134*, *135*, 135–6, *136*
epiglottis 99–100, *100*, 112–13, *112*
epiphyseal plate (growth plate), in a
    bone 28, *29*
epiphysis (end) of a bone 28, *29*
epithelial tissue (epithelium) *17*,
    17–18
erythrocytes (red blood cells) 85–6,
    85, *86*
    in birds 169
erythropoiesis 85, 86
erythropoietin 79, 86, 122
Eustachian (auditory) tubes 73, *74*,
    99, 112, *112*
excretion 107
    by the kidneys 130–1
    by the urinary system 122
exfoliative cytology 144
exocrine glands 18
exocytosis 8
expiration (exhalation) 105
expiratory reserve volume 105
extension, of a joint 42, 44
external abdominal oblique muscles
    49, *50*
external acoustic (auditory) meatus
    30, *30*, 73, *74*
external ear 73, *74*
external intercostal muscles 105
external nares 98, *98*
external urethral orifice 140, *142*
extracellular fluid (ECF) 11
extraocular muscles 47–8, *48*
extrinsic muscles 46
    of the forelimb 50–1, *51*
    of the hindlimb 52
    of the eyeball 71
eyelashes, conditions associated with
    72
eyelids *71*, 71–2
eyes 67–73
    extrinsic muscles 71
    fields of vision 68, *69*
    formation of an image 72–3, *72*
    muscles 47–8, *48*
    structure and functions *69*, 69–71
eyesight, of birds *164*, 164–5

facial expression, muscles of 47
facilitated diffusion 6
faecal incontinence 119
faecal retention 119
faeces 119
false pregnancies 146
family (classification) 3
fascicles 22
fat cells 20, *20*
fats (lipids)
    digestion of 116–18
    in food 116
    metabolism in the liver 120
fatty acids 14, 118
fatty tissue 19, 20
'fear, fight or flight' syndrome 82–3
feathers
    dust and pathogens 162
    structure of 161, *163*
    types and functions 161–2, *163*
feeding tube, care with guinea pigs
    182
femur 39–40, *40*
ferret (*Mustela putorius furo*) (order
    Carnivora)
    dentition 185
    digestive system 185–6, *187*
    morphology 184–5
    musculoskeletal system 185, *185,
    186*
    reproductive system 186, *187*
    urinary system 186, *187*
fertilisation 10, 146–7, *147*
fibrinogen 85, *85*, 87
fibroblast cells 20, *20*
fibrocartilage 20
fibrous connective tissue 19, 20
fibrous joints 41–2
fibrous proteins 15
fibula 40, *40*
filtration *13*
fish (class) 3
fish (Teleost group) 200–3
    circulatory system 202
    digestive system 202
    gill system 202, *203*
    integument 202
    live-bearing species 203
    mouth brooders 203
    musculoskeletal system 200, *200*
    osmoregulation 202
    reproductive patterns 202–3
    respiratory system 202, *203*
    special senses *201*, 202
    swim bladder 200–1, *201*
    urinary system 202
flagella *6*, 8
flexion, of a joint 42, 44
flight muscles 159
'floating' ribs 35–6, *36*
fluid balance in the body 11, 12–13,
    13–14
fluid mosaic model *6 see also*
    phospholipid bilayer
fetus *see* embryo and fetus
follicle stimulating hormone (FSH)
    78, 79, *82*
food boluses 108, 109, 112–13, *113*,
    115
footpads 154–5, *155*
foramen 29
foramen magnum 63
foramen ovale 93
forebrain 60–1, *60*

forelimb
    bones of *27*, 36–9
    muscles of 50–2
fossa 29
frontal bone 30, *30*
frontal sinus 98, *99*
frusemide (diuretic) 128
functional residual capacity 105
fur 153–5

gall bladder 107, 116, 119
ganglion cells 71
gaseous exchange, in the alveoli
    101–2, *102*
gastric dilation and volvulus (GDV)
    113
gastric juices 113, 117–18
gastric pits 114, *115*, 117
gastrin 79, 117
gastrocnemius muscle 53, 54, *54*
general anaesthetics, and the
    blood–brain barrier 62
genus (classification) 3
gerbil (*Meriones unguiculatus*)
    (Myomorph) 178
    dentition 179
    digestion 179–80
    digestive system 179–80
    morphology 179
    physiological and behavioural data
    188
    reproductive data 189
    reproductive system 180, *180*
    sexual differentiation 180
germ cells, division 8, 10–11
gestation period 146
gingival membrane 109
gizzard, in birds *169*, 170
glandular tissue, types and functions
    17, 18, *19*
glaucoma 71
gliding/sliding joints 42, 44
globular proteins 15
glomerular capsule 124, *125*, *126*
glomerulus (Bowman's capsule) 124,
    125, 126
    functions of 126, *126*, *127*
glottis (larynx) 99–100, *99, 100*
    muscles of 48
glucagon 78, 81
glucocorticoids 79, 82
gluconeogenesis 82
glucose 14, *14*, 118, 119
glucosuria 81, 127
gluteal muscles 52, *53*
glycerol 14, *14*, 110
glycogenesis 81, *81*
glycogenolysis 81, *81*, 83
goblet cells *17*, 18
Golgi apparatus (or body) 5, *6*, 7
gonadotrophin releasing hormone 79,
    81, *82*
Graafian follicles 139, *141*, 143
gracilis muscle 53, *54*
granulocytes (granular leucocytes)
    85, *85*, 86, 86–7
greater curvature 113, *115*
grey matter (cerebellum) 61
grey matter (cerebral cortex) 60
grooming 109
growth hormone 78, 79
guinea pig (*Cavia porcellus*) 178
    dentition *181*, 181–2
    digestive system 181–2, *182*

    need for vitamin C 182
    morphology 181
    physiological and behavioural data
    188
    reproductive data 189
    reproductive system 183
    sexual differentiation 183
    skeletal system 181
    urinary system 184
gums 109
gustation (taste) 66, *68*

haemoglobin 14, 86
haemopoiesis 27, 85
haemopoietic organ 95
haemopoietic tissue 19, 20
haemorrhage 86
haemothorax 103
hair 153–5
hair follicles 153, *154, 155*
hamster (*Mesocricetus auratus*)
    (Myomorph) 178
    dentition 179
    digestion 179–80
    digestive system 179–80
    morphology 179
    physiological and behavioural data
    188
    reproductive data 189
    reproductive system 180, *180*
    sexual differentiation 180
hamstring muscles 52, *53*
hard palate 109, *109*
Haversian systems (in bone) 21, *21*
head, muscles of 47–8
hearing, birds 165
heart 24, 87–90
    birds 168
    cardiac cycle 88–9
    circulation of blood through 88–9,
    89
    conduction system 89–90, *89*
    'hole' in 93
    position in the thorax 103
    reptiles 191
heart auscultation, in Chelonians 191
heart chambers 88
heart murmur 88, 93
heart valves 88, *89*
heart wall, layers 88
heparin 87
hepatic artery 92, 93, 119, *120*
hepatic portal system *92*, 93
hepatic portal vein 92, 93, 118, 119,
    120
hepatic vein *92*, 93, 119, *120*
hepatocytes 119, *120*
Hering-Breuer reflex 105
hermaphroditism, in fish 202
hibernation, Chelonians 191
hindbrain 61, *60*
    respiratory centres 105
hindlimb
    bones of 39–41
    muscles of 52–4
hinge joints 44
hip bones 39, *39*
hip dysplasia in dogs 39, 54
histamine 86, 87
histiocytes 96
hock joint *41, 43*
    muscles of 54
    point of 40, *43*
'hole' in the heart 93

homeostasis 11, 14, 60
    functions of the blood 84
hormones 15
    changes during oestrous cycle 144
    chemistry 77
    endocrine glands which produce
        78–9
    of lactation 142
    production and transport 18
    response produced 77
    sources of 77, 79
    stimuli for secretion 77
    transport 84
humerus 37, *38*
    fractures of 37
humoral immune response 96
hyaline articular cartilage *41*, 42
hyaline cartilage 20, *21*
    model for bone 28, *29*
hyoid apparatus 31, *32*, 99–100, *100*
hyoid bone, attachment of tongue
        109
hypaxial muscles *48*, 48–9
hyperadrenocorticalism 82
hyperglycaemia 81, 127
hyperparathyroidism 80
hyperthyroidism 80
hypertonic fluids 12
hypertrophy of muscles 46
hypodermis (subcutaneous layer)
        152–3, *152*
hypothalamus 60, 78, 79, *82*
hypothyroidism 80
hypotonic fluids 12
hypovolaemic shock 13
Hystricomorph rodents 181–4

ICSH (interstitial cell stimulating
        hormone) 78, 79, 81–2
ICF (intracellular fluid) 11
ileocaecal junction 116
ilium 39, *39*
immune response
    non-specific 96
    specific 96
immune system 85, 86–7
    defence systems 96
    functions of the blood 84
immunoglobulins 85, 96
implantation 146–7
incisive bone *30*, 31, *31*
incisor teeth 31, *31*, *110*, 110–11
    overgrowth in rodents 179
infection
    enlargement of lymph nodes 95,
        96
    protection against 86–7
    signs in popliteal lymph node 54
inflammatory processes 86–7
inflammatory response 96
infraspinatus muscle 51, *51*
ingestion 107
inguinal hernia 50
inguinal ring 50, *50*
inner ear *74*, 74–5
inorganic compounds in the body 11,
        13–14
insectivores 4
inspiration (inhalation) 105
inspiratory reserve volume 105
insulin 78, 81
integument 5
intercalated discs, in heart muscle *22*,
        23

intercalated neurons 58, 65
intercellular products 17
intercostal muscles 36, 105
intercostal nerves 105
internal abdominal oblique muscles
        50, *50*
internal intercostal muscles 105
interphase before meiosis 10, *10*
interphase before mitosis 8, *9*, 9
interstitial cell stimulating hormone
        (ICSH) 78, 79, 81–2
interstitial fluid 11, 17
interventricular septal defect 93
intervertebral disc 33, *34*
intestinal juice 117, 118
intestinal wall, structure of 116, *117*
intracellular fluid (ICF) 11
intramembranous ossification 28
intraocular pressure 71
intravenous injections 109
    birds 169
intrinsic muscles 46
    of the forelimb 51–2, *51*, *52*
    of the hindlimb 52–4
intubation 99
    birds 167
    rabbits 177
invertebrates 3
ions 13
iris 69, 70
iron 14, 86
iron-deficiency anaemia 86
ischium 39, *39*
islets of Langerhans 81
isometric contraction 46
isotonic contraction 46
isotonic fluids 12

Jacobsen's organ
    lizards 194
    snakes 198
jaw muscles 47, *47*
jejunum and ileum 107, *107*, *108*,
        116
joint capsule *41*, 42
joints 41–4
jugular veins 92, *92*

keratin 15
keratinised stratified epithelium 18
kidney disease 131
kidneys 122–31, *123*
    blood supply *124*, 124
    formation of urine 124–31
    macroscopic structure *123*,
        123–4, *124*
    microscopic structure 124, *125*
kingdom (classification) 3

lachrimal gland *71*, 72
lacrimal bone 30, *30*
lactase 118
lactation 142–3
lacteals 94, 116, *117*, 118
lagomorphs 4, 173–8
large intestine 107, *107*, *108*, 113,
        118–19
laryngeal paralysis, in dogs 100
larynx (glottis) 99–100, *99*, *100*
    muscles of 48
lateral (definition) 4, *4*
lateral canthus *71*, 71
lateral line system, in fish *201*, 202
latissimus dorsi muscle 51

left atrioventricular (AV) valve 88, *89*
leg and foot, of birds *160*, 160–1, *161*
lens 69, 71
    formation of an image 72–3, *72*
lesser curvature 113, *115*
leucocytes (white blood cells) 85, *85*,
        86, 86–7
ligaments 20, 29
    in synovial joints *41*, 42, *43*
limbus 71
linea alba aponeurosis 49–50, *50*
Linnaeus, Carl 3
lipases 118
lipids 7, 14, *14*
lips 108–9
live-bearing fish 203
liver 107
    functions 119–20
    hepatic portal system *92*, 93
    structure 119, *120*
lizards (suborder Sauria) 193–7
    autotomy 194
    cardiovascular system 194, *195*
    digestive system 194, *195*
    handling 194
    integument 194
    respiratory system 194
    sexual differentiation 196, *197*
    skeleton 193, *194*
    special senses 194
    urogenital system 196, *196*
loop of Henle 123, 124, *125*, 127,
        127–8
lumbar vertebrae *27*, 32
    shapes of 34, *35*
lungs *100*, *101*, 101–4, *103*, *104*,
        104–5
    division into lobes 102, *103*
luteinising hormone (LH) 78, 79, *82*
lymph fluid 11, 118
lymph nodes 94, 94–5, *95*, 96
lymphatic capillaries 94
lymphatic ducts 94, *94*, 96
lymphatic system 94–6
lymphatic tissues 95
lymphatic vessels 94, *94*
lymphocytes 85, *85*, *86*, 87, 95
lymphoid tissue 85
lysosomes 5, *6*, 7, 8, *8*
lysozymes 7, 8

macrophage cells 20, *20*, 87, 96
magnesium 13, 14, 85
malar abscess 110
malocluded teeth
    guinea pigs 181
    rabbits 176, *176*
maltase 118
Mammalia (class) 3, *4*
mammary glands 142–3, *142*, 153
mandible (lower jaw) 31, *31*, 108,
        109
mandibular glands 111, *111*
mandibular symphysis 31, *31*, 42
manubrium 24, 36, *36*
mass movements, in the large
        intestine 119
masseter muscle 47, *47*
mastication 108
    muscles of 47, *47*
mating
    cat 139
    dog 139
maxillary sinus 98

medial (definition) 4, *4*
medial canthus *71*, 71
median plane 4, *4*
mediastinum 24, *25*, 88, *101*, 102, 103–4
medulla oblongata *60*, 61
medullary cavity 27, *28*
meiosis 8, 10–11
membranous cochlea *74*, 74
membranous labyrinth *74*, 74
membranous semicircular canals *74*, 75
membranous vestibule *74*, 75
meninges 62, *62*
menisci, in a joint cavity *41*, 42, *43*
mesaticephalic skull shape 32, *33*
mesentery *25*, *26*, 113
metabolism 15, 107
metacarpus 38, *38*
metaphase of mitosis *9*, 9
metaphase I of meiosis *10*, 11
metaphase II of meiosis *10*, 11
metatarsus 40, *41*
microvilli 116, *117*
micturition (urination) 132
midbrain 61, *60*
middle ear 73, *74*
milk, composition of 143
milk fever in cows 57
milk (temporary) teeth 110–11
mineral salts, in plasma 84–5
mineralocorticoids 79, 82
minerals, in the body 13–14, 27
mitochondria 5, *6*, 7
mitosis 7, 8–9, *8*
mixed nerves 58
molars *110*, 110–11
molecules 13
monocular vision (2D) 68, *69*
monocytes 85, *85*, *86*, 87
monoestrous cycles 145
monogastric digestion 113
monoglycerides 118
monorchid 137
monosaccharides 118
motor nerves 58
motor units 46
moulting
    birds 163
    of hair 153
mouse (*Mus musculus*) (Myomorph) 178
    dentition 179
    digestion 179–80
    digestive system 179–80
    morphology 178
    physiological and behavioural data 188
    reproductive data 189
    reproductive system 180, *180*
    sexual differentiation 180
mouth breathing 99
    diving birds 166
movement, synovial joints 42–4
mucous membranes *17*, 18
multicellular glands 18, *19*
multiparous females (dog and cat) 139
muscles
    anatomy 46, *46*
    attachments 46, *46*
    belly 46, *46*
    contraction 45–6, *45*
    heads 46, *46*

neuromuscular junction 56
    shapes 46, *46*
    sheath 22
    tissue types and functions 17, 21–3, *22*
    tone 46
    responsible for respiration 104–5
muscular system 5
myelin sheath 23, *23*, 56
myeloid tissue 85
myocardium 22, 88, 89
myofibrils 22, 45, *45*
Myomorph rodents 178–80
    coprophagia 180
    dentition 179
    digestion 179–80
    digestive system 179–80
    reproductive system 180, *180*
    sexual differentiation 180
myosin (thick) filaments 45, *45*
myxoedema 80

nasal bone 30, *30*
nasal cavity 98, *99*
nasal chambers 30, 98
nasal mucosa (smell) 66–7
nasal septum 30
nasal turbinates (conchae) 30, 98, *99*
nasolachrimal duct *71*, 72
nasopharynx 99, *99*, 109, *112*
neck muscles 48
nephrons 123
    structure of 124, *125*
nerve fibres 23, *23*
    and muscle contraction 45–6
nerve impulses 56–7
    generation of 57–8, *58*, *59*
nerves, classification of 58–9
nervous system 5, 56–66
nervous tissue 17, 23, *23*
neuroglial cells 56, 62
neurohypophysis 78, 79–80
neurons 23, *23*
    size of 56
    structure 56–7
    variations in shape 56, *57*
neutrophils 85, *86*, 86
nictitating membrane (third eyelid) *71*, 72
    in birds 165
night vision 70
nodes of Ranvier 56
non-myelinated nerve fibres 56, *56*
non-self cells, destruction of 96
noradrenaline (norepinephrine) 79, 82–3
nose breathing *112*
nose, structure and functions 98–9, *98* see also nasal
nosepad 98, *98*
nucleoli 6, 7
nucleus 5, *6*, 7
    division by mitosis 8–9, *9*
nucleus pulposus 33, *34*
nutrients, transport 84

occipital bone 30, *30*
oesophagus 107, *107*, *108*, 113
oestrogen 78, 81, *82*, 82, 143
oestrous cycle 143–6
    changes in ovary and reproductive tract 143–4
    functions of 143
    hormonal changes 144

phases in the bitch *144*, 144–5
phases in the cat (queen) 145–6, *145*
phases of 143
olecranon 37, *38*
olfaction (smell) 66–7
olfactory bulbs *60*, 61, *61*, 67, 98
olfactory nerves 31
olfactory region of the nose 98
omentum, greater and lesser *25*, *26*, 113
optic chiasma 60, *61*
optic disc *70*, 71
oral cavity (mouth, buccal cavity) 107, 108–9, *109*
orbit 30, *30*, 67
order (classification) 3
organ of Corti *74*, 74, 75
organelles 5, *6*, 7–8
organic compounds 11, 14–15
organogenesis 149
organs 5, 17
oropharynx 99, *99*, 109, 112
os penis 28, 137–8, *139*
osmoregulation 84, 122, 128–30
osmosis 11, 12, *13*
osmotic pressure 12
    of the blood 85
ossa coxarum (hip bones) 39, *39*
ossification 28, *29*
osteocytes 21, *21*
otitis externa, in dogs and cats 73
otoliths 75, *75*
ova 8
oval window *74*, 74
ovarian artery 141
ovarian hormones 78
ovaries 77, *77*, 78, 81, *82*, 139, *141*
    cell division within 10
    changes during oestrous cycle 143
ovariohysterectomy 140
over extension, of a joint 44
oviducts (Fallopian tubes) 139–40, *140*, *141*
oviparous reproduction, reptiles 190
oviviparous reproduction, in fish 203
ovoviviparous reproduction, reptiles 190
ovulation 143
    induced 145
    spontaneous 145
oxygen, diffusion across pulmonary membrane 101
oxygen transport 84
oxyhaemoglobin 86
oxytocin 78, 70

pacemaker *89*, 90
palmar 4, 5
palpebral reflex 72
pancreas 77, *77*, 78, 80–1, 107, 116
pancreatic duct 116
pancreatic hormones 78
pancreatic juice 117, 118
panting in dogs 109
papillae, on the tongue 109
paranasal sinuses 98–9, *99*
parasitic infestation 86–7
parasympathetic nervous system 66, *67*, 68
parathormone 78, 80, *80*
parathyroid glands 77, *77*, 80
parathyroid hormones 78
parietal bone 30, *30*

parotid glands 111, *111*
parotid nodes 95, *96*
parthenogenesis
    in fish 202
    in lizards 196
patella *27, 28, 40, 43,* 52
patella reflex 66
patella slippage, in dogs 40
pectineotomy, to help hip dysplasia 54
pectineus muscle *53,* 54
pectoral muscles 51, *51*
pelvic cavity *24, 25, 26*
pelvis 39, *39*
penis
    dog 137–9
    functions of 137
    structure of 137–9, *138*
    tomcat 139
pepsin 117, 118
perching reflex, birds 161
pericardial cavity 24
pericardium 24, 88
perilymph *74,* 74
periodontal membrane 109
periosteum 21, *21*
peripheral nervous system 56, 63–6
peristalsis 113, *113,* 115, 116, 119
peritoneal fluid 25
peritoneum 25, *26*
permanent dentition *110,* 110–11
pH 14
    balance in the body 14, 84
phagocytic cells *see also* macrophages
    blood cells 96
    in lymph nodes 95
phagocytosis 7, 8, *8,* 20, 86, 87
phalanges 38–9, *38*
pharynx 48, 99, *99,* 107, 109, *109,*
    112–13, *112*
pheromones 153
philtrum *98,* 109
phospholipid bilayer 5–6, *6*
phosphorus 14
photoreceptor cells 67, *70,* 70–1, 72
phylum (classification) 3
physiology (definition) 3
pia mater 62, *62*
pinna 73, *74*
pinocytosis 8
pituitary gland 60, *61,* 77, *77*
pituitary hormones 78, 79–80
pivot joints 44
placenta 93, 149
plane/gliding joints 42, 44
plantar (definition) *4,* 5
plasma 11, 84–5, *85*
plasma membrane 5–6, *6,* 7–8
plasma proteins 11, 85
platelets *85, 86,* 87
pleural cavities *101,* 102–3
pleural membranes 24, *25*
    types of *101,* 103, *104*
pneumothorax 103
polymerisation 14
polymorphonucleocytes (PMNs) 86
polyoestrous breeding season 145
polypeptides 14
polysaccharides 14
pons *60,* 61
popliteal node 95, *96*
    signs of infection 54
pores, in the cell membrane 6, *6*
posterior (or caudal) (definition) *4, 4*
posterior chamber 71

posterior pituitary gland 78, 79–80
postsynaptic membrane 57
potassium 13–14, 57, *59,* 85
preen gland 159
pregnancy 81
prehension 108
premolars *110,* 110–11
prescapular nodes 95, *96*
presynaptic membrane 56
primates 4
progesterone 78, 81, *82*
prolactin 78, 79
prophase of meiosis *10,* 11
prophase of mitosis 8–9, *9*
prophase II of meiosis *10,* 11
prostate gland *134, 135,* 137, 139
proteases 118
proteins (polypeptides) 14–15, *15*
    digestion of 116–18
    in food 116
    metabolism in the liver 120
    structure 14–15, *15*
    synthesis 7
    transport 7
prothrombin 85, 87
protraction, of a limb 42
proximal (definition) 4, *4*
proximal convoluted tubule 124, *125*
    functions of 126–7, *127*
psittacosis 162
pterygoid muscles 47
pubic symphysis 42
pubis 39, *39*
pulmonary artery 90
pulmonary circulation 88, 90, *92,*
    93, *92,* 93
pulmonary membrane 101
pulmonary pleura *101,* 102
pulmonary valve 88, *89*
pulmonary vein 91
pulp cavity 109
pulse 89, 109
pupil *69,* 70
    size control, in birds 165
pupillary reflex 72
Purkinje cell *57,* 61
Purkinje fibres *89,* 90
pyloric sphincter 115, *115*
pyloric stenosis 115
pyothorax 103

quadriceps femoris muscle 52

rabbit (*Oryctolagus cuniculus*) (order
    Lagomorpha)
    digestion 177–8
    digestive system 174–7, *175*
    handling of 173
    morphology 173
    physiological and behavioural data
        188
    position of scrotum 177
    reproductive data 189
    reproductive system *177,* 177–8,
        178
    respiratory system 177
    skeleton 173–4, *174, 175*
    teeth 176–7, *177*
    urinary system *177,* 177
    young 178
radius 37, *38*
rat (*Rattus norvegicus*) (Myomorph) 178
    dentition 179
    digestion 179–80

digestive system 179–80
    morphology 178
    physiological and behavioural data
        188
    reproductive data 189
    reproductive system 180, *180*
    sexual differentiation 180
rectum 107, *107, 108,* 119
rectus abdominus muscles 50, *50*
reflex arcs 65–6
rehydrating fluids, tonicity 12
relaxin 81
renal failure, chronic 131
renal nephrons, processes occurring
    in 124, *127*
reproductive organs 25, *26*
reproductive system 5, 134–50
    birds *171,* 171–2
    female 139, *140*
    male 134–9
    male dog *134*
    tomcat *135*
reproductive tract, changes during
    oestrous cycle 143–4
reptiles (class Reptilia) 3
    cardiovascular system 190
    classification 190
    digestive system 190
    handling 191
    heart 191
    integument 191
    renal portal system 191
    reproduction 190
    respiratory system 190
    skeletal system 190
    thermoregulation 191
    urinary system 190
residual volume 105
respiration (pulmonary ventilation)
    control of 105
    definition of 98
    external 98
    in birds *167,* 167–8
    internal (tissue) 98
    mechanics of 104–5
    muscles responsible for 104–5
respiratory centres, hindbrain 105
respiratory definitions 105
respiratory rate, dog and cat 105
respiratory region of the nose 98
respiratory system 5, 98–106
    in birds 165–8, *166*
reticulocytes 86
retina 67, *69,* 69, *70,* 70–1
    formation of an image 72, *72*
retraction, of a limb 42
rhinarium *98, 98*
rhythmic segmentation 115, *116,*
    116, 119
ribosomes 5, *6,* 7
ribs 24, 34–6, *36*
right atrioventricular (AV) valve 88,
    89
right lymphatic duct 94, *94*
rodents (order Rodentia) 4, 178–84
rods (light sensitive cells) *70,* 70
rostral (definition) 4, *4*
rotation, of a joint 42, 44
round window *74,* 74

saccule *74,* 75
sacral plexus 65
sacral vertebrae *27,* 32
    shapes of 34, *35*

sacroiliac joint 34, 39, 39
sacroiliac ligament, stretching during parturition 34
sacrum 34, 35
sagittal crest 30
saliva 108, 111–12
salivary enzymes 108
salivary glands 107, 111, 111–12
    birds 170
salt gland, marine birds 171
sarcomeres 45, 45
sartorius muscle 53, 54
scapula 36–7, 37
Schwann cells 23, 23, 56, 56
Sciuromorph rodents 180–1
sclera 69, 69
scrotum 134, 135, 135, 136
sebaceous glands 152, 153
secretin 79, 118
selectively permeable membrane 5–6, 6
semilunar valves 88, 91
semimembranosus muscle 52, 53
seminal fluids 139
seminiferous tubules 135, 136
semi-permeable membranes 12, 13
semitendinosus muscle 52, 53
senses, specialised 66–75
sensory nerves 58
serotonin 56
serous fluid 24
serous membranes 24–5
Sertoli cells 135
serum 85, 85
sesamoid bones 38, 39
sex hormones, adrenal 79, 82
sexual reproduction 134–50
shedding of hair 153
shoulder joint 37
sight 67–73
simple diffusion 6
simple epithelium 17, 17
sinoatrial node (pacemaker) 89, 90
sinuses 28
    frontal 30
    paranasal 98–9, 99
skeletal (striated) muscle 22, 22, 45–55
skeletal system 5, 27–44
    functions 27
skeleton
    appendicular 27, 28
    axial 27, 28, 29–36
    of birds 159–61, 160
    splanchnic 28
skin, structure and functions 151–3, 152
skin colour, in relation to hair colour 152
skin glands 153
skin infections, fish 202
skull, birds 159–60, 161
skull bones 29–32, 33
skull shapes
    dog 31–2, 33
    domestic cat 31
'slipped disc' 33
small intestine 107, 107, 108, 113, 116–18, 117
smell (olfaction) 66–7
    in birds 165
smooth (unstriated, involuntary, visceral) muscle 22, 22
snakes (suborder Serpentes)

cardiovascular system 197
digestive system 198, 199
fangs 198, 198
integument 197
respiratory system 197, 199
sexual differentiation 198–9
skeleton 197, 198
skull 197, 198
special senses 197
tongue 198
urogenital system 198
vertebrae 197, 198
sodium 13–14, 84
    entry into cells 6
    osmoregulation 129–30, 130
    transmission of nerve impulses 57, 59
soft palate 99, 99, 109, 109, 112, 112
somatic cells, division 8
somatic sensory and motor nerves 59
somatostatin 78, 81
somatotrophin 78, 79
sound, perception of 75
sound production 48, 100, 109
spaying 140
special senses 66–75
species (classification) 3
specific immune response 87, 96
spermatogenesis 135
spermatozoa 8, 135, 137
sphenoid bone 30, 30
sphincter muscles 46
spinal canal 32, 34
spinal cord 32, 59
    structure 63, 64
spinal nerves 64, 64–6
spinous process (on vertebra) 32, 33, 34, 35
splanchnic skeleton 41
spleen 95–6, 113–14
squamous cells 17, 18
sternal ribs 35, 36
sternebrae 36, 36
sternum 24, 35, 36, 36
steroids 7, 82
stifle joint 28, 40, 43
stomach 107, 107, 108, 113
    functions of 113
    gastric emptying 115
    muscular movements 115
    simple 113
    structure of 113–14, 115
    wall, structure and function 114–15, 115
stomatitis ('mouth rot') in Chelonians 191
stratified epithelium 17–18, 17
stretch receptors, respiration control 105
striated muscle 22, 22
structural systems of the body 5
subclavian veins 92, 92
sublingual artery 109
sublingual glands 111, 111
sublingual vein 109
sublumbar hypaxial muscles 52
submandibular nodes 95, 96
succus entericus 116, 118
sucrase 118
superficial (definition) 4
superficial cervical nodes 95, 96
superficial inguinal nodes 95, 96
supraspinatus muscle 51, 51

supratrochlear foramen (dogs) 37, 38
surgery, use of linea alba for sutures 50
suspensory ligaments 69, 70
sutures (joints) 31, 41–2
swallowing (deglutition) 99–100, 112, 112–13
    muscles for 48
sweat glands 153
swim bladder, fish 200–1, 201
sympathetic nervous system 66, 67, 68
synapses 23, 23, 56–7
synaptic cleft 56–7
synarcosis 50
synarthroses 42
syncitium 10, 11
synovial (tendon) sheath 46, 47
synovial fluid 42
    in a bursa 46, 47
synovial joints 41, 42–4
    ranges of movements 42
    types and properties 44
synovial membrane 41, 42
systemic circulation 88, 90, 91–3, 92
systems, in the body 17
systole 89, 90

tail, vertebrae in 34, 35
tapetum lucidum 70, 70, 72
tarsus 40, 41, 43
taste, sense of (gustation) 109
    in birds 165
taste buds 66, 68, 109
taxonomy 3–4
tears 72
teeth 109–11
    dog 31
    eruption times 111
    function 109–10
    shapes and features 110, 111
    structure 109
    types and functions 110, 111
telophase of mitosis 9, 9
telophase I of meiosis 10, 11
telophase II of meiosis 10, 11
temperature control 84, 109
temporal bone 30, 30
temporalis muscle 47, 47
temporomandibular joint 31, 108
tendons 20, 29
tensor fascia latae muscle 52, 53
terrapins see Chelonians
testes 10, 77, 77, 79, 81–2, 134, 135, 136, 135–7
testicular descent 136–7
testicular hormones 79
testosterone 79, 81–2, 135
thalamus 60
thermoregulation 84, 109
thigh muscles 52–4, 53
third eyelid 71, 72
thoracic cavity 24, 24, 25, 101, 102–4, 103, 104
thoracic duct 94, 94, 96, 118
thoracic vertebrae 24, 27, 32
    shapes of 34, 35
thorax, muscles of 49, 49
thrombocytes (platelets) 85, 85, 86, 87
thymus 96
thyrocalcitonin 80, 80
thyroid glands 77, 77, 80
thyroid hormones 78

thyrotrophic/thyroid stimulating
    hormone (TSH) 78, 79, 80
thyroxin 78, 80
tibia 40, *40*
tidal volume 105
tissue fluid 11, 122
tissues of the body 5, 17–23
    types 17
T-lymphocytes 87, 96
tongue muscles 48
tongue 48, 99, 109, *109*
tonicity (osmotic pressure) 12
tonometer 71
tonsils 112
tortoises *see* Chelonians
total lung capacity 105
touch (sense of) in birds 165
trachea 99, 100
tracheal collapse, in dogs 101
tracheal ducts 94, *94, 96*
transcellular fluid 11
transmitter substances 56
transversus abdominis muscles 50, *50*
trapezius muscle 50, *51*
triceps brachii muscle 51, *52*
tricuspid valve 88, *89*
tri-iodothyronine 80
trochanter 29
trochlea 29
trunk, muscles of 48–50, *48*
tubercle 29
tuberosity 29
tunica vaginalis *136*, 137
turbinates 30, 98, 99
turtles *see* Chelonians
tympanic bulla 30, 73
tympanic cavity 73
tympanic membrane (ear drum) 30,
    73, *74, 75*

ulna 37, *38*
ultrafiltration 11, 126, *126*
umbilical cord 149
unconditional reflex 66
ungulates 4
unicellular glands *17*, 18

urates 170
urea 130
ureters *122, 123, 124*, 131
urethra
    female *122*, 131
    male *134, 135*, 137, *138*
    male dog 131
    tomcat 131–2
uric acid 170
urinalysis 132–3
    in reptiles 191
urinary system 5, 122–33
    birds 170, *171*
    functions of 122
    parts of 122, *122*
urinary tract, blockage by uroliths or
    calculi 131
urination (micturition) 132
urine
    constituents of 130–1
    formation by kidneys 124–31
urogenital system 25, 122, *123*
urolithiasis 131
uropygial gland 159
uterine artery 141
uterine tubes (oviducts) 139–40, *140,
    141*
uterus *140*, 140
utricle *74, 75, 75*
uvea 69, *69–70*

vagina *140*, 142
vaginal epithelium, changes during
    oestrous cycle 143–4
vasopressin 80
veins 90, 91
venepuncture 91
    lizards 194
venous circulation 92, *92*
ventral (definition) 4, *4*
ventricles 88, *89*
ventricular system (brain) 61–2, *62,
    88, 89*
venules 91
vertebrae
    basic plan 32, *33*

formula for *27*, 32
    joints between 33, 34
vertebral column
    functions of 32
    muscles of 48–9, *48*
    regions of *27*, 32
vertebrates 3
vestibule 142
vestibulocochlear nerve (VIII) *74*, 75
villi (sing. villus) 116, *117*, 118
visceral muscle 22, *22*
visceral peritoneum 113
visceral sensory and motor nerves
    59
visceral systems of the body 5
vital capacity 105
vitamin C, guinea pigs' requirement
    for 182
vitamin K 87
vitreous humour *69*, 71
viviparous reproduction, in fish 203
vocal folds 100
vocal ligaments 100
vomiting 112, 113
    three types of 115
vulva *140*, 142

waste products, transport 84
water
    content of the body 11–13
    intake required 13
    loss, control of 128–9, *129*
    loss, due to sickness or injury 13
    loss, normal 12, 13
    medium for body's biochemical
        reactions 11
white matter (cerebellum) 61
white matter (cerebrum) 60
wings, structure of *160, 161, 162*

xiphoid cartilage 36, *36*
xiphoid process 36, *36*

zygomatic bone (zygomatic arch,
    cheekbone) 30, *30*
zygomatic glands 111, *111*

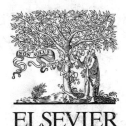

ELSEVIER

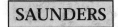 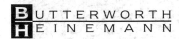

SAUNDERS   Mosby   BUTTERWORTH HEINEMANN

VETERINARY PUBLISHERS OF CHOICE FOR GENERATIONS

For many years and through several identities we have catered for professional needs in veterinary education and practice. Saunders and Mosby, the leading imprints for veterinary medicine and Butterworth Heinemann, the leading imprint for veterinary nursing, are now part of Elsevier. Our expertise spreads across both books and journals and we continue to offer a comprehensive resource for veterinary surgeons and veterinary nurses at all stages of their career.

As the leading international veterinary publisher we take our role seriously and are proud to offer, in association with the British Veterinary Nursing Association, two annual bursaries to veterinary nursing students. For further details please contact BVNA at www.bvna.org.uk .

To find out how we can provide you with the right book at the right time, log on to our website, www.elsevier-health.com or request a veterinary catalogue from the Marketing Department, Elsevier, 32 Jamestown Road, Camden, London NW1 7BY, tel: +44 20 7424 4200, emarketing@elsevier-international.com.

We are always keen to expand our veterinary list so if you have an idea for a new book please contact either Mary Seager, Senior Commissioning Editor for Veterinary Nursing/Technology (m.seager@elsevier.com) or Joyce Rodenhuis, Commissioning Editor for Veterinary Medicine (j.rodenhuis@elsevier.com). We can also be contacted at Elsevier, The Boulevard, Langford Lane, Kidlington, Oxford OX5 1GB, UK (tel +44 1865-843000).

 Have you joined yet?
Sign up for e-Alert to get the latest news and information.

Register for eAlert at www.elsevierhealth.com/eAlert Information direct to your Inbox